# LOSING YOUR SIGHT

## Ellen Daniels

D0513122

ROBINSON
London

Constable Publishers
3 The Lanchesters
162 Fulham Palace Road
London W6 9ER
www.constablerobinson.com

First published in the UK by Robinson,
an imprint of Constable & Robinson Ltd 2001

A copy of the British Library Cataloguing in
Publication Data is available from the British Library.

ISBN 1-84119-327-5

Printed and bound in the EU

*This book is dedicated to my son Laurence
and my daughter Belinda
for their constant support.*

# Contents

# *Acknowledgements*

I would like to acknowledge the following people for their support and assistance in the preparation of this book:
Mike Lancaster, Director of External Relations, RNIB; Mr J.F. Giltrow-Tyler BSc., Principal Optometrist, Bristol Eye Hospital; Optometric Adviser, Department of Health; Hilary Todd, Independent Editor; Marion Jackson MA Cantab Modern Languages, Teacher of French and Religious Education (Retired) at Croydon High School, GDST; Peter Coombs LSIAD, graphic designer; Debbie Maizels CBiol., MIBiol. medical illustrator; Roger P. Phillips BVSc. (QLD), MRCVS, veterinary surgeon; John F. Brumell ACIB, computer expert and Kathleen Starr, retired civil servant.

## Note

The names given to individual cases are fictitious and in some instances small details have been altered to preserve anonymity, but the cases are all factual and known to me personally. In most of them, permission to quote has been readily given; some, however, have died; and a very few are no longer traceable.

I have largely abandoned the use of the formal him/his or her in favour of the simpler 'them' or 'their', which is in common spoken usage.

# Foreword

Nearly two million people in the UK have a severe sight problem – around 1 in 30 of the population. We are all familiar with the apparently confident and independent blind person we see regularly – on the bus or train or out and about at the local shops, quite possibly with the support of a guide dog, but seemingly coping well. However, the majority of people who have a serious sight loss are elderly, quite often stuck at home, and very dependent on others for support, including organisations like the Royal National Institute for the Blind (RNIB) and local societies for blind people.

Research shows that it is sight that is the sense people fear losing most. Ellen Daniels and many like her have overcome their disability to the extent of leading as normal a life as a sighted person would expect. Yet Ellen is not typical of blind people. Apart from raising a family on her own for much of her life – since the time she became registered blind – she has given very valuable service in counselling, particularly to others with sight loss, and above all has written this compelling firsthand account of life without sight, for the benefit of others, like myself, who can never fully understand the difficulties blindness causes.

Blind people are people first, and blind second, yet for many, however independent the minority may be, they still face problems of becoming fully integrated into their local community. Hopefully this book will help to further the task of raising awareness of the needs of these people with uncorrectable sight loss, and create more understanding of how we can all break down some of the barriers for blind people, and indeed for those with other disabilities as well. The book is peppered with cameos from the lives of real blind people, helping us to get a firsthand feel of the extra dimension sight loss brings.

Many people who have sight loss, and perhaps those facing the onset of serious sight loss in later life, will find Ellen's book a practical guide of great value, at a time of confusion and difficulty. I sincerely hope it will also be read by sighted people who want to find out more about what it is like to live without sight. If it does this, as I'm sure it will, it will have succeeded doubly and served its purpose. Those of us, like myself, who have experienced a close relative, possibly a parent, losing their sight in later life, will find it invaluable.

In my father's case, although he became registered blind, in his view he just couldn't see as well as he had done years before, while undeniably finding it almost impossible to accept he couldn't do simple things he had treasured, like reading the daily horse racing form! I suspect many of the readers of this book will have friends or relatives who are or have been in a similar position, and the practical and common-sense guidance Ellen provides will give support in time of stress.

At a more specialist level, I commend Ellen's chapter on counselling, particularly in her own case as a blind counsellor of people with sight problems. This is an area which has had little written about it, and I'm sure Ellen's experience and insight will provide much food for thought.

This book is about coping with blindness, yet coping is not a word that springs readily to mind in the case of Ellen Daniels herself. In her life, and in writing this book, she has proved that 'coping' is an inadequate term to describe her. While in no way belittling the pain and distress sight loss brings, I believe Ellen's book will be an inspiration to others for whatever reason they have chosen to pick up her book.

This task is ably assisted by Ellen's writing, based on her own experience and the real lives of people who live with blindness every day.

One of the most fundamental tasks undertaken by RNIB is to raise public awareness of the needs of blind people, and those who have a serious or uncorrectable sight loss.

Mike Lancaster

*Director of External Relations*
*Royal National Institute for the Blind*
*March 2001*

# Preface

The starting point for this book is the eye condition which has affected me from birth. It was unknown then and remained unrecognised in me until, when I was 24, it was diagnosed by consultant ophthalmologist Joseph Minton, as Retinitis Pigmentosa. He was in the process of writing a book about the condition and used photographs of my eyes to illustrate it. Some years later, I learned that my condition was caused by a recessive gene, common to both my parents, who were carriers, passing it on only to me out of their five children. We knew of no other case in either family within living memory.

I was registered blind at the age of 35. Nine years later, widowed and with two dependent children, I was offered a place at the Rehabilitation and Assessment Centre at Torquay (Manor House), then run jointly by the Department of Employment and the RNIB. This was a three-month residential course for men and women of working age – mostly men – who hoped to retrain and continue to support their families. Within two weeks of my arrival, I found myself chosen as captain of the current group of students: I had no idea that this was to be a major turning point in my life.

My role was that of intermediary between residents and staff, and it was while listening to the students that I discovered the terrible consequences for many of them of losing their sight. Their experiences brought home to me the need (at that time unrecognised) for professional support and counselling, particularly in personal and emotional matters, for people losing their sight. Shortly after leaving the Centre, I was offered a post with a Social Services Day Care Division. The 19 years I spent there enabled me to learn about disabilities other than blindness; but it was a dead-end job, and I felt spurred on by my Torquay experience to seek the academic qualifications I had so far lacked.

It took me six years to obtain an Open University degree, by which time my sight had deteriorated to the extent that I was using a cane, so I trained with my first guide dog. I also took an initial course in counselling, following which I acquired two diplomas in public speaking. These opened doors for me to give lectures and run workshops on Understanding Blindness for students and professional bodies, including staff in teaching hospitals.

At this point, the Open University asked me to undertake some staff training in Disability Awareness and Understanding Blindness, and then to become one of their counsellors for disabled applicants in the London area. A local voluntary association for the blind, knowing my interest in counselling, offered me regular employment with them.

For several years I was a team leader on special weekend courses for visually impaired students in their first year with the Open University, men and women of widely differing ages and backgrounds and with a variety of visual impairments. What they had in common was a determination to take a degree and make something of their lives, despite their sight loss. Their resolution is repeated in countless blind and partially sighted people who would like to make positive choices in life, despite their disability.

I now work for four charities for the blind, for two of them as a counsellor, one as a staff trainer and one as a speaker, whilst continuing to extend my counselling work. Recently I took a London University course in Pastoral Care and Counselling, which I have found invaluable.

I have also been involved with preparing local primary school pupils to accept into their midst visually impaired children who are being integrated into mainstream schooling.

The main body of my work is now, however, with older blind and partially sighted people – their ages ranging from 16 to 96 – and with their families. I have learned of appalling traumas, as well as great courage, and witnessed how much damage and suffering are caused through society's failure to understand the emotional and social effects of sight loss. It would be very helpful if training programmes for all professions could contain a module on Understanding Blindness.

My purpose in writing this book is to make those who encounter blind people more aware of the needs of this part of the community, and how they may be more fully integrated into that community.

# *Introduction*

Most sighted people misunderstand what the word 'blindness' covers and, without direct contact with the world of the blind, fail to grasp the important fact that not many blind people are in total darkness. Around 96% of those who are severely visually impaired have some residual vision, varying from a limited ability to read, but with no peripheral vision, to a faint and perhaps fleeting perception of light.

This book is largely aimed at fully sighted people who have had no experience or explanation of visual impairment. It is written in order to help them understand what it means to be blind, to explain why the behaviour of visually impaired people may be misinterpreted and how best the needs of these people can be met.

The book is also directed towards those, both professional and non-professional, who come into contact with and/or care for visually impaired people and their families. I hope that it will help to create an understanding of those who cannot see very well, and so make life easier for them and all concerned with them.

# 1

# *Communication*

Much of this chapter is concerned with the forms of communication that are open to the blind and the partially sighted – and those that are not.

## Interpersonal Communication

Communicating with others is a basic human need, and one of the most fundamental ways of achieving that communication is through eye contact.

### Loss of Eye Contact and Resulting Isolation

Eye contact is the most fundamental means of communication between all mammals, with the exception of those living in dark places, such as moles, bats and whales. It is essential for the promotion of psychological, social and emotional well-being. A great deal of information can be exchanged and intentions read at this first contact with each other's eyes.

Humans are at the top of this mammalian animal chain and eye contact is an important part of our daily life and social intercourse. When, in 1997, the President of Russia, Boris Yeltsin, received the Prime Minister of Great Britain, Tony Blair, the President's first words were, 'You have good eyes.' Already, a primary means of communication had been established between them.

Looking directly into a person's eyes can reveal unspoken feelings and emotions. We can tell whether someone is sad or unwell, hurt or angry; we can see a look of longing or a far-away look; and to glimpse two people looking lovingly at one another, even across a room, is a clear indication of something special between them.

This information, however, may only be passed on to those who not only have eyes, but have sight. Occasionally a sighted person will wear dark glasses in order to prevent others from reading their emotional condition – the wearer's feelings and thoughts remain effectively concealed. A similar situation occurs when someone suffers from a condition such as a squint. In this instance, lack of focus prevents eye contact being secured and the sighted person is therefore unable to read what is behind the eyes.

Just as a dog when coursing a hare will stare at it and put it into a trance, so a hypnotist will use his skills with eye contact to put his client into an hypnotic state, the one using the transmission of fear with the intention to kill and the other using a state of mesmerism during clinical treatment. Yet eye contact offers us more than the ability to transmit or receive information from other people non-verbally – it can also be the means of discovering a truth. It gives us a nasty shudder when something nice is being said in a polite situation, but a glance at the eyes shows them to be cold or dismissive. At that point, we know we have to believe the eyes and not the ears. Eye contact gives us a very important means of recognising the intention or mood of the person who is communicating with us. Those who are deprived of this means of communication miss a part of life which it is impossible to replace. This is true in every sphere of life, which the following examples illustrate.

*In a Students' Workshop*
When I am running a training workshop for professional people on Understanding Blindness, I put them into a situation where half of them are under blindfold. A suitable but controversial topic is given for discussion. After a short hesitation, somebody is bursting to say something in favour of or against the motion and a heated discussion usually begins. It is then important to watch what happens, which is very revealing. The people under blindfold want to join in the discussion, but find this very difficult because they are not given the opportunity to do so by the rest of the group. This is because the eyes of the sighted participants are not drawn to the eyes of those under blindfold. If the discussion

is allowed to go on for long enough, some of the blindfolded students will be seen to be leaning back out of the group. The sighted students continue the discussion without them.

On occasion, a very brave blindfolded student will bang his fists on the table or shout from sheer frustration, 'Will you please let me get *my* point across!' The others are usually stunned and a bit confused, because they have no idea that the argument is being conducted only between themselves.

In a discussion with the whole group following this exercise, it becomes apparent to the participants that eye contact is crucial to human relationships and discourse. Equally, lack of eye contact causes feelings of isolation, rejection and frustration.

Teachers of any subject must be aware that a sight problem could be the reason why a student is not joining in with the rest of the group. All students have to be given the opportunity to get their point across in a group discussion. Most of us have seen a small child put both their hands over their eyes and announce, 'Can't see me!' Visually impaired people often feel like this when with a group or a crowd of other people: it is as if their sight loss has caused them to disappear.

*Within the Family*
A painful illustration of what is going on can be seen in an ordinary family, where one of the

members is suffering sight loss and is in a residential home – let us say the widowed mother. The son collects her in his car for Sunday lunch, and the rest of the family is also invited. Affection is lavish. Mother is seated in the best chair at the head of the table for the meal, and it is here where the heartbreak begins.

The family all talk to one another, not deliberately ignoring the mother, but because they are unable to make eye contact with her, they do not draw her into their conversation. All she can do is to sit and listen, trying very hard to remember that the family does not intend to be hurtful. Like the young child, mother feels that she has been made invisible.

## In the Residential Home

A further illustration can be the depression caused by lack of eye contact in places such as homes for the elderly blind, where residents are inclined to give up more easily because of their age. Quite unable to make contact with anyone other than those who are sitting next to them, there is a longing from time to time to talk to somebody else.

## In the Workplace

The situation in offices and factories where there may be one blind person can also be very difficult. The demands of the job are not the source of the problem, for the employee will have been properly trained, value their job and do it as well as anyone else. It is in the everyday, more social part, of the working environment where blind people feel the most isolated – in the canteen or the cloakroom, or even in the office or on the factory floor itself. As in the experiment which I described earlier, so often the person with no ability to make eye contact 'disappears' from the group. A guide dog can help enormously to alleviate the problem, because people will want to come and talk to the dog from time to time. Some people, however, may not wish to have a dog and many employers are reluctant to have a dog in the workplace.

*Body Language*

Another problem which comes from a similar source is a blind person's inability to read other people's body language: while his body language can be read, he is unable to do the same. This is significant whatever the situation: the nod of the head, the raised eyebrows, the shrugging shoulders, the smile or the extended hand, the look cast across the room to someone else. Everyone else in that situation is able to read the body language exhibited by the person without sight, who may feel isolated and in certain situations very vulnerable, because he is observed but unable to observe. Imagine the plaintiff in a court case being unable to see: his obvious anxiety and nervousness could be misinterpreted to his disadvantage.

Similarly, a blind person's reactions to a situation may appear inappropriate to the occasion. This is illustrated by two examples from my experience as a counsellor. In the first, Robert was taken to Russia by a group of sighted friends. On a sightseeing trip, they inadvertently entered a church during a funeral service. Robert was devastated at finding himself suddenly ushered out of the church by his friends, who had been shocked by the sight of the body resting in an open coffin. Robert had been unaware of their distress and of the solemnity of the service being conducted – he had therefore not been able to respond appropriately to the situation. For many years afterwards, he regretted what must have appeared to be his lack of sensitivity, to those unaware of his visual impairment.

In the second example, Fred lived for many years with the humiliation of having been asked to leave the army during the war. This was because he was apparently stupid, clumsy, slow to react and insensitive to changing situations. Long afterwards, it was discovered that Fred had an eye condition which caused a very restricted field of vision. Therefore the cause of his inappropriate reactions was his eye condition, not stupidity. However, this early rejection and the stigma which he attached to it during the intervening years caused low self-esteem and eventual deep depression.

\*   \*   \*

Eighty per cent of information is taken in through sight. Therefore, without sight the other senses have to be relied on far more and intuition becomes more important. This does not happen automatically, as sighted people sometimes imagine. The remaining senses – touch, hearing, taste and smell – do not improve as a result of sight loss, but need to be used more effectively.

The importance of body language is evident everywhere to the sighted person. In any social situation, careful observations may be made which illustrate this point. Try observing a couple in a bar. It is evident from the subconscious matching of their body language whether their relationship is intimate or just beginning. In other situations, such as a therapeutic setting, the therapist may deliberately contrive to match the body language of his patient in order to create an empathy. For the visually impaired, these means of building a relationship are denied.

## *Verbal Communication*

As we have seen, eye contact is very important in the animal kingdom and in particular to the human animal, where this means of communication can have a bearing on all the emotions. However, unlike the rest of the animal world, human beings have language, and verbal communication has developed between people of like race or tribe in hundreds of different ways throughout the world.

From the day of their birth, most healthy babies are able to make all the sounds contained in languages everywhere, but within a short time they will eliminate the sounds which are not heard in their native tongue. Within 18 months or so, they can successfully shape those sounds into the words they hear from people with whom they come into contact. They have learned to do this by watching the facial movements made by people who speak to them, particularly their mothers.

Try holding a young baby securely under its arms so that its feet are on your lap and the baby is facing you. She will enjoy feeling her feet for a few minutes. Now talk to her. Tell her a story. You'll find the baby will be watching your face intently, and you will see that she is moving her mouth and lips in an attempt to imitate what you are doing. As she makes the sounds she hears around her, she is just beginning to shape those sounds, gradually learning to use all her organs of articulation, especially the lips and the jaw. Eventually the baby is able to form the words she understands and learns to speak her own language. She has done so by watching and listening, adding together what she sees with what she hears.

In this way, we all grow up through childhood and into our adult years looking at a person's face, particularly the lips, when listening to what someone is saying. Consequently, most fully sighted people learn some degree of lip-reading without realising what they are doing. Hence when Aunt Mary says, 'Just a minute dear, I can't hear you, I've lost my glasses', it is not as funny as it seems to be, because she needs to read your lips to understand exactly what you are saying to her.

Even in the cinema, our eyes focus upon the faces of those on the screen, and so it is with the television or in the theatre and in ordinary social conversation. It is therefore very important when speaking to someone who is unable to see to use clear speech. It is very difficult to understand someone if they are mumbling, hardly using their lips, speaking with their back to you, or in a bad light, and even more difficult if they are speaking too quickly.

So it is easy to understand why the telephone is an ideal means of communication for people who are unable to see. Now, both parties in the conversation are on the same level. Neither can see the other and, provided they both speak clearly, they are able to communicate freely, without disadvantage to the one who cannot see.

## Alternative Means of Communication

Our world is dominated by the printed word – from signs in the street to labels in the home, from billboards to bank statements; it takes little imagination to see how disadvantaged – and even at risk

– blind people are. In the second part of this chapter, I shall examine the alternative means of communication that are available to them.

*Braille*

Most sighted people believe that all the visually impaired can read Braille. This is quite untrue, but for those who can master it, Braille does provide a valuable form of communication.

Braille consists of a system of raised dots, creating symbols which form a kind of print and are read by the fingertips. It was invented by Louis Braille (1809–1845). At the age of three, he badly damaged an eye with a sharp tool picked up in his father's workshop; the subsequent infection led to the loss of sight in both eyes. Before he was twenty, he had been introduced to and perfected a system of printing for blind people using various permutations of just six raised dots.

Blind and partially sighted children are taught Braille from an early age and it becomes their accepted form of print throughout their lives. They may reach a speed of 200 words a minute. During their educational years, they will learn a contracted form of Braille, enabling a great deal more to be put on to one page. Modern developments in printing have greatly improved the quality of the print. There are also Braille forms of shorthand, of musical notation and of mathematical symbols.

A disadvantage of this method is that Braille

books and magazines are large, heavy and clumsy and all Braille is expensive to produce. There is a national library for the blind in Stockport, where a good supply of books can be obtained. From this library, books – each consisting of several volumes – are sent out free of charge. Each volume is approximately 15 inches long, 10 to 12 inches wide and 1 to 2 inches thick. A long, popular novel such as *The Shell Seekers* by Rosemary Pilcher, for example, comes in 15 volumes – not an easy book to read on the train or under the drier at the hairdresser's. Some books may be purchased from the National Library (which normally lends them) and from the Royal National Institute for the Blind at a heavily subsidised rate for blind readers.

In the home, Braille symbols are useful for the purposes of identification. Labels can be made quite easily. In addition, cookers and washing machines can have Braille controls.

## Written Braille

Writing Braille can be a problem. For those who can afford to buy one, there is a Perkins machine, sometimes mistakenly referred to as a Braille typewriter. For this, one has to get used to imagining the Braille symbols as if they were opened out and laid horizontally. There are three keys either side of the space bar in one horizontal line. As the correct keys are depressed, so the probe goes into the special manila paper and the dots come through on the other side. This is the means by which most Braille is printed by sighted people for the benefit of those unable to see. It is difficult to find sighted people who are willing to learn Braille in order to produce documents. Recently, a successful and greatly valued scheme was introduced into some prisons, where prisoners are taught and encouraged to do this work.

There is another, cheap, method of putting plastic dots onto thin paper which is not meant to be kept but to be destroyed after use. This is therefore used for things like television and radio programme magazines, although this method is only used by large organisations such as the RNIB, who have special machinery for this purpose.

Without the aid of machinery, one has to use a stylus, with the manilla paper attached to a board by a special frame. Because one works from the back of the paper, the writer has to think backwards, beginning on the right, and printing the Braille the opposite way round. When the paper is released it can be read from left to right. This might be fun for some people to do, particularly those who enjoy word games! However, if you are writing a shopping list, making notes or writing a letter to someone else who reads Braille, it needs a great deal of thought and concentration, although of course it comes naturally to people who have never learned anything else.

Technology is gradually coming more and more

to the aid of those who cannot see. For example, there is a small machine which uses a combination of Braille, synthesised voice and computer technology. With an input of Braille, the machine will read the messages back, but it is extremely expensive and at present has limited use outside the offices of professional people.

Of course, there are many who like to keep their independence and struggle to use Braille as much as they can. However, it is by no means easy for those who have learned to read print and used it through early adult life to embark later upon something which needs entirely different skills. Furthermore, certain physical conditions such as arthritis, poor circulation, diabetes and hand and arm injuries, diminish the sense of touch. Similarly, the results of all kinds of manual work, including housework, may cause an insensitivity in the fingers which prevents the effective use of Braille.

## Moon
Another form of raised print, rather like large capital letters with bits missing, is called Moon. Although some elderly people enjoy learning and reading from it, it is difficult to produce and only a limited choice of reading material is available.

## Tape Recorders and Cassettes
There is nowadays a wide variety of radios and

tape recorders for listening and recording in mono or stereo sound. The visually impaired can therefore keep up with current events and enlarge their horizons through listening and reading, in the same ways that other people do. The *Radio Times* is available on tape, as are local newspapers and selections from some Sunday papers. There is also a whole variety of specialist tapes, from catalogues to magazines, from official publications to works of literature.

Equally, where writing would be the usual medium, many people now send letters to friends and families abroad by speaking the letter onto a cassette audio tape which can be posted. Very often the recipients will reply in the same way, and so contact between sighted and unsighted people may be maintained. However, despite these advances in technology and availability, the frustration felt by a blind reader when a tape spills into the machine, for example, can be unbearable. It is almost impossible to recover the tape and rewind it without breakage when relying only on your sense of touch – and it usually happens at the most exciting part of the story!

### Audio Tapes

Some of the first advances in the world of technology brought about the RNIB's talking book service. At first, the machine on which the tapes were played looked like a small piece of furniture and was certainly not portable. Now the machine for these same tapes is relatively small, easy to operate and very popular amongst its users.

The RNIB library has a vast range of books on every topic, including text books for blind students. This service is available to all registered blind people, who receive their books post free. The machine has to be rented, which some Social Services departments will pay for. Local libraries today have a good selection of taped books – as they do of books in large print. The tapes are available to everybody, including sighted people, so there may be a long wait for the more popular ones.

## *Identifying Documents*

In addition to the usual tape recordings, it is now possible to attach a strip of audio tape to a piece of card and, by passing it through a machine called a VOX-COM recorder, to play back letter headings and other short pieces of information. These are useful in the identification of documents, compact discs and personal items, once more enabling someone previously able to read print to preserve just a little more of their independence.

## *Television and Radio*

Television can be a fine aid to the visually impaired; closed circuit television, where print can be enlarged black on white or white on black, can be extremely helpful, particularly in the office or the educational setting. In the home, television also has its uses for visually impaired people. This is because in real life, panoramic views are not accessible to those with a restricted field of vision. The television screen reduces this panorama to a size where everything is in proportion and the viewer can see the whole scene, be it a sheep dog trial or the Houses of Parliament on the banks of the River Thames. This point is seldom recognised even by the viewer, who may be unaware that the television screen is in fact a means which brings him a greater feeling of being part of the world outside. With some visually impaired people, a smaller – say, 14-inch-screen, may yield greater clarity than a larger one.

But TV has its limitations, since it is essentially a visual medium. By contrast, radio scores for blind people because it reaches us through sound alone, and through the imagination. The characters in radio plays all have distinctive voices; one has only to listen to *The Archers* to realise how carefully it is cast! Radio uses sound effects to create atmosphere and supply the scenery.

*Keyboard Skills*
Training in keyboard skills has been the norm for many years in the education of visually impaired children, and is now a part of the curriculum throughout the nation's primary schools. Young people so trained, and anyone who has undergone

a business course, will have acquired the skill of touch typing. Should such people lose their sight, they will have a great advantage in that they will still have the means of communication with sighted people through print.

Some people who lose their sight later in life may find that they are able to learn touch typing at this stage. For people of working age, help with such skills may be obtained through a variety of organisations, particularly the RNIB and Action for Blind People (see Chapter 9 for contact details for these organisations). However, for a variety of reasons, many will not be able to learn to touch type, especially, for instance, when blindness comes together with a physical disability.

It is now possible to purchase a computer with a synthesised voice, enabling more people who become visually impaired to continue working by using a computer. A disadvantage here is that such computers are often complicated to use and are extremely expensive, although more advances are occurring almost on a daily basis. Technology marches on!

# 2

# *The Eye and What Blind People See*

The effects of visual impairment cannot be fully understood without a basic knowledge of the eye and how it works. Only then will comprehension of the cause, or causes, of the malfunction and disorder be possible. This applies, of course, as much in human physiology as it does in the fields of electronics and engineering. So often, when the doctor or ophthalmologist refers to things which sound familiar, such as cataracts or the iris, few of us know exactly what these are or how they function. It is common for people to imagine that a cataract is a kind of membrane which causes cloudy vision and has to be removed, or even that the iris serves only to give colour to the eye. Neither is true.

In the face of complicated conditions such as Retinitis Pigmentosa or Optic Atrophy, the patient and carer urgently need to understand the terminology used. For this reason, I have included a simplified description of the parts of the eye and how sight is formed in this chapter, together with an explanation of some of the more commonly known eye conditions which cause malfunction. I hope that this will help to further the understanding of those who are personally connected or professionally involved with visually impaired people.

## The Eye

Nature has adapted the eye to ensure it is used to its maximum efficiency in the environment in which it has to work, whether human, animal, bird, fish or insect. In cats, for example, during the daytime the pupil will look like a narrow slit, resembling curtains which have been drawn together to shut out the excess light. The owl, on the other hand, will appear to have had the curtains drawn back at night time when it is hunting, in order to admit the maximum amount of light. The hawk, hunting his prey at constantly changing distances, must have an eye which will rapidly change focus. Likewise, the human eye has adapted to give us colour vision, an awareness of dangers around us and acute vision with which we can manage fine tasks.

In the human eye, the near-spherical eyeball bulges at the front, where light is allowed to enter. There are two oblique and four straight muscles attached to the outside of the eyeball, which enable movement up, down, left, right and slightly rotating, ensuring that the maximum field of vision is obtained without the need to move the head. The white of the eye, which completely covers the outside of the eyeball and is known as the sclera, is tough and strong. The bulge in the front, also tough and strong, is known as the cornea. The cornea is quite clear and is commonly known as the window of the eye.

Beneath the sclera lies the choroid, which is dark in colour and carries the blood vessels which nourish the eyeball. Where the choroid bends away from the cornea at the front of the eye, a coloured curtain which we call the iris surrounds the pupil. The colour of the iris varies from person to person, ranging from the deepest brown to the palest blue, and in some cases it is colourless. The pupil is an opening, the size of which is controlled by circular and radiating muscles contracting or expanding in the iris. In bright light, the pupil is small, whilst in dim light the iris causes the pupil to dilate to allow the maximum amount of light into the eye.

At the back of the eye, to receive the picture of the outside world, lies the complex retina. Its millions of cells detect, code and process the image, converting it into nervous signals, before sending those signals to the brain via the optic nerve. The retina and optic nerve are an extension of the brain, and it is in the latter's visual cortex that the signals are decoded and become what we recognise as sight. The optic nerve is therefore a conduit for information from the eye to the brain. Where the optic nerve leaves the eye, a 'blind spot' can be found in the field of vision, because no retinal tissue overlies the point where it exits the eye. To a doctor or optometrist, the optic nerve head is the most distinctive feature to be found on examining the inside of the eye.

The macula, exactly in the centre of the back of the eye, is that part of the retina with the most densely packed receptors, giving us our most acute vision.

Inside the eye is the flexible crystalline lens which, by altering its shape, enables us to refocus between near and distant objects, for example, from reading to television. This fine focusing ability is lost in middle age and later life. This lens lies just behind the iris. The lens, iris and back of the cornea are bathed in nutritious aqueous humour, which is produced in the ciliary body at the back of the root of the iris. Aqueous humour is drained from the eye through small channels which lie in the angle formed by the back of the cornea and the root of the front of the iris. If too much aqueous humour is produced, or the exit channels are blocked, the pressure inside the eye increases, causing damage to the nerves; this is known as glaucoma. Behind the lens is the jelly-like, transparent vitreous humour, the function of which is to fill out the bulk of the eyeball (see Figures 1A and 1B).

When an image passes through the eye, it is inverted and back-to-front by the time it reaches the retina, but the brain has the capacity to re-erect the image. The eyes are the instrument of sight, working in a similar way to a sophisticated digital camera, but it is the brain which interprets the signals and produces the sensation we recognise as sight.

Many people have a minor abnormality of the eyes which, whilst impeding the sight, may easily be overcome by wearing corrective lenses, usually prescribed by an optometrist. For example, when the eyeball is too long or too short from back to front, the person will be short- or long-sighted; when the cornea is not a section of a true sphere, the picture may be slightly distorted by being indistinct in one direction and strikingly clear in another. Although these conditions in themselves are not considered too serious, bear in mind that spectacles and contact lenses should be regularly checked and replaced as the condition changes (see Figure 2).

Overwork and reading in a bad light, or of course wearing the wrong lenses, may eventually lead to a worsening of the complaint, headaches or eyestrain. Updating the prescription, adopting better working habits, or improved lighting may alleviate many of these problems. About 4% of

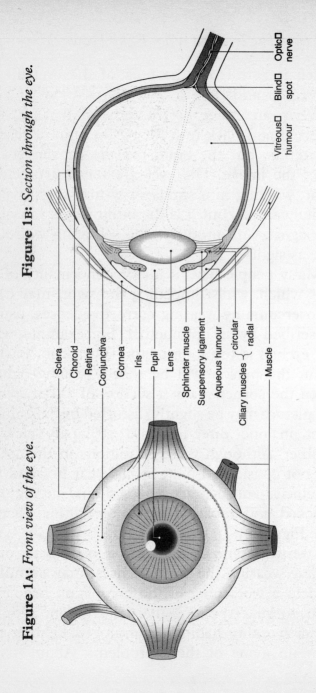

**Figure 1A:** *Front view of the eye.*

**Figure 1B:** *Section through the eye.*

Sclera
Choroid
Retina
Conjunctiva
Cornea
Iris
Pupil
Lens
Sphincter muscle
Suspensory ligament
Aqueous humour
Ciliary muscles { circular
radial
Muscle

Optic
nerve

Blind
spot

Vitreous
humour

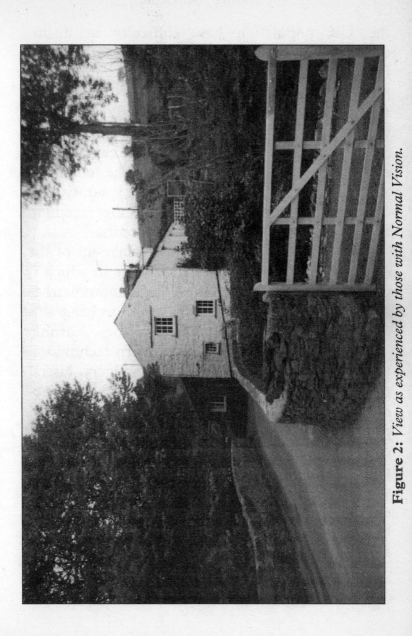

**Figure 2:** *View as experienced by those with Normal Vision.*

the UK population have difficulty in distinguishing colours, with around 10 times more men being affected than women. Defects range from mild confusion of greens and browns, through to the inability to recognise red from green and/or yellow from blue. A few people are very severely affected and are only able to distinguish difference in levels of luminance, rather like looking at a colour film on a black and white TV set. Colour deficiency is caused by a fault in the reception and processing mechanisms of the retina.

Once we understand the basic make-up of the eye, we can begin to investigate ways in which it can malfunction. Ophthalmologists, optometrists and orthoptists spend many years studying this precious part of the human physiology, learning skills required to treat it with modern techniques, technology and medication. Microsurgery, lasers, ultrasound, improved drugs, sophisticated spectacle and contact lenses are used today and produce excellent results. There are far fewer cases of blindness at birth, because of better treatments and drugs and a greater understanding of the administration and withdrawal of oxygen to premature babies, who are at risk of blindness if the oxygen they receive is not administered properly.

# Some Common Eye Conditions Explained

## *Diabetic Retinopathy*

This is a disease of the eye which affects some of the 2% of British people who suffer from diabetes. Approximately half of diabetics will at some point experience changes in the back of the eye. As the diabetes progresses, many do not deteriorate beyond showing minor 'background' changes, but in some cases leakage from minute blood vessels occurs, which may affect central vision. More serious complications include haemorrhages of blood into the vitreous humour, retinal detachment and sometimes total loss of sight. However, in most cases, sight-threatening changes can be treated, using a laser, which is done by an ophthalmologist in a hospital. Diabetics should have frequent eye examinations from an optometrist, ophthalmologist or through an accredited photographic screening programme, since treatment in the early stages may prevent irreversible sight loss (see Figure 3).

## *Disciform Macular Degeneration*

One of the major causes of sight loss, this condition is most common in people over the age of 75. The central part of the retina at the back of

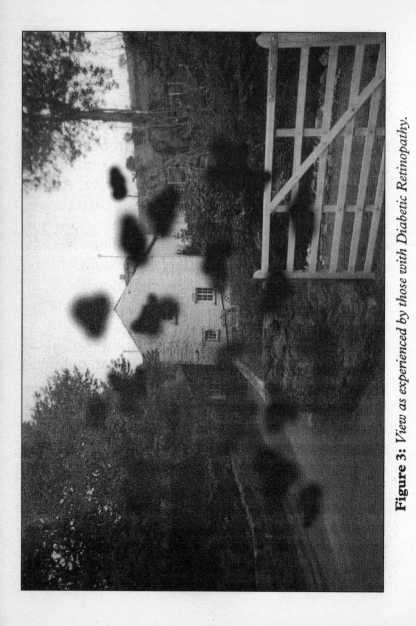

**Figure 3:** *View as experienced by those with Diabetic Retinopathy.*

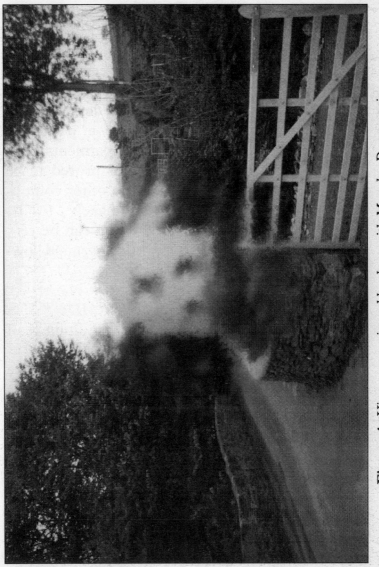

**Figure 4:** *View as experienced by those with Macular Degeneration.*

the eye takes care of the central detail of what we see, and is known as the macula. It is, however, prone to degeneration with age: blood vessels can start to leak and cause scarring, which irreversibly damages the vision. The central vision becomes blurred and distorted, whilst the peripheral vision remains intact. Vision loss can be sudden, sometimes occurring over a period of weeks or a few months. Various treatments have been tried, but nothing to date has proved to be really effective. Where there are no other complications, the whole sight is unlikely to be completely lost. The peripheral vision can be very useful sight and can be supported by good low-vision aids (see Figure 4).

### Age-Related Macular Degeneration (ARMD)

Again, those who suffer from this condition tend to be elderly. Loss of vision is usually not as marked, nor as sudden as in those who have disciform vision loss. The changes tend to be slow and insidious, occurring over a number of years. Sufferers at first tend to complain of the inability to see detail, for instance newsprint, or people's faces. ARMD is not treatable at present, but can easily be confused with and complicated by cataracts, as it is not uncommon for the two to occur together. It is important to distinguish between them, because surgical treatment is available for cataracts. ARMD is caused by degenerative changes in the retinal cells, which pick up the light and cease to function as they age.

*Posterior Vitreous Detachment and Floaters (PVD)*
This is a condition likely to affect people in later life (over the age of 55). It is a degenerative condition where the vitreous humour, the jelly-like substance which fills the cavity at the back of the eye, shrinks and falls slightly forward. As it does so, it stimulates the retina, so affecting the nerve cells and the optic nerve. The person concerned sees flashing lights, often coming towards them. There may also be thickenings in the vitreous fluid, which produce the effect of irregular black shapes passing before the eyes, which are usually referred to as floaters. Occasionally a cobweb effect is caused. But although at first these flashing lights, floaters and cobwebs may be frightening and even nauseating, the flashing lights usually disappear with time and the floaters and cobwebs become much less noticeable.

A PVD in itself is harmless, but on very rare occasions the jelly-like fluid diminishes, pulling at the retina, where a hole or even a detachment is created. Flashes of light, together with floaters and shadows around one eye, will indicate that emergency treatment is needed and the person should go straight to hospital (see Figure 5).

*Hemianopia*
This also usually affects people in the upper age

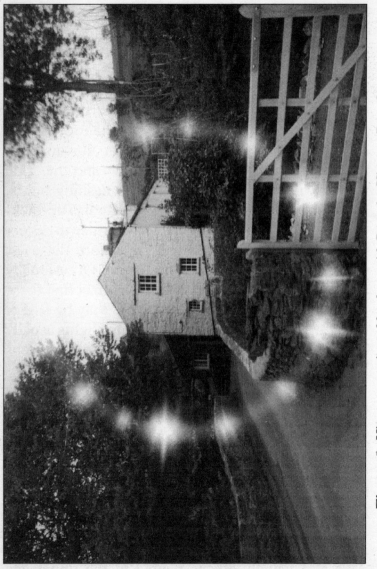

**Figure 5:** *View as experienced by those with Posterior Vitreous Detachment.*

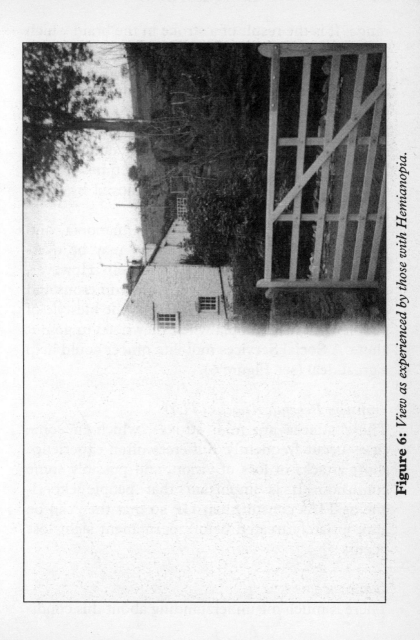

**Figure 6:** *View as experienced by those with Hemianopia.*

range. It is the result of a stroke in the brain which obliterates the vision in the same half of each eye, either both left or both right. For the sufferer, there is therefore not even the full range of vision of one eye, since each eye is restricted in the same way. At first the person's orientation and balance become severely affected and there is a feeling of insecurity. Reading becomes difficult and sometimes impossible, but television may still be enjoyed by some people with this condition.

It is possible to get used to hemianopia, and potential dangers within the home may be overcome with a little adjustment and help. However, the hazards in the outside world are numerous and particular attention must be paid to the lifestyle of people with hemianopia when they need to go out alone. A Social Services mobility officer could help a great deal (see Figure 6).

## Transient Ischemic Attacks (TIA)

These attacks are mini strokes, which in some cases occur frequently. Sufferers often experience short attacks of loss of vision, and possibly some confusion. It is important that people experiencing TIAs consult their GP so that they can be appropriately treated before permanent sight loss occurs.

## Cataracts

There is much misunderstanding about this condition, usually because few people know how the eye is constructed. A cataract is an opacity within the crystalline lens, which prevents a clear image from reaching the retina at the back of the eye. The image becomes increasingly blurred as time goes by, and the opacity becomes more dense or increases in size. Cataracts may be found in any age group, from congenital cataracts, where the infant is born with the condition, through middle to old age, and may be in one or both eyes.

At one time, to be told one had cataracts was a sentence to blindness in later life. Nowadays, for those who have no other serious eye condition, the removal of the lens – replaced by an artificial lens for which the patient is carefully measured in advance – may be undertaken on a day-surgery basis at the local hospital. It can be less distressing or painful than having a tooth removed at the dentist's. In the case of double cataracts, one on each eye, one cataract will be removed at a time, the second after an interval of six months or so.

In Gordon's case, before surgery the cloudiness had become quite dense, even to the point of total sight loss, and the joy on recovery of the sight is clearly understood. He was depressed, frightened and even anguished before the operation, when he could see only light and dark. His words to me were, 'Before I had the first operation I could see nothing around the windows in my room, just a patch of cloudy light to tell me where the windows

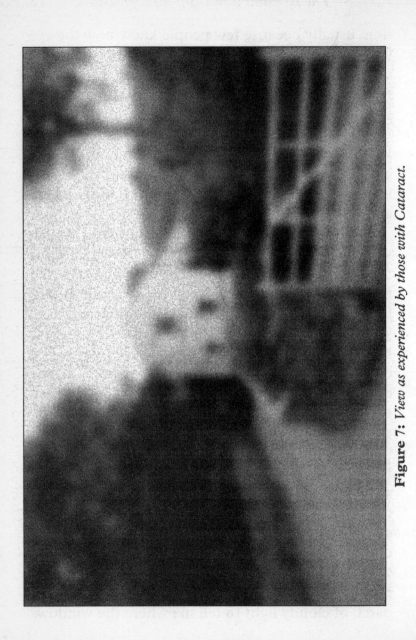

**Figure 7:** *View as experienced by those with Cataract.*

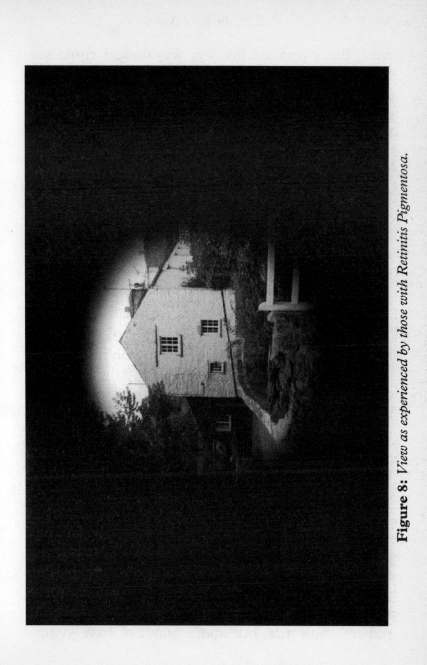

**Figure 8:** *View as experienced by those with Retinitis Pigmentosa.*

were, but when the first eye was done I could see the curtains, the window and the walls and when the second eye was done, I could see the pattern on the curtains, on the walls and the carpet too.' Gordon was a very happy man.

There is little hope, however, of this joyous outcome when there is another serious condition present in the eyes. A surgeon will perform the operation, but it may only improve things slightly and for a little while. In these cases, there is often great disappointment and the patient will need considerable support (see Figure 7).

## Some Inherited Eye Conditions

The above eye conditions are some of the better known and more commonly dealt with in the field of work with blind and partially sighted people. All these conditions severely impair the sight, which becomes in one way or another distorted. However, there are many other eye conditions, rare and obscure, which may be caused by accident, infection, illness, tropical disease, parasites, trauma and inherited conditions.

## Retinitis Pigmentosa (RP)

This is one of the best-known inherited eye conditions. It worsens over time and may initially present itself as an inability to see well at dusk and in the dark. People are usually affected from puberty onwards, but some may not have symptoms until their twenties. The visual field is gradually lost peripherally, leading to severe mobility problems as tunnel vision becomes increasingly evident. Later in adult life, the remaining central vision may be affected by cataracts and, unfortunately, some RP sufferers lose their vision entirely. If the condition is not too severe, the cataracts may be removed, which will improve the central vision for quite a long time. This is not, however, always possible. (The case study of George in Chapter 3: Barriers, is a classic example of this condition at its worst.)

Deposits of pigment appear on the periphery of the retina and later in the central areas. The blood vessels which serve the retina begin to shrink and optic atrophy occurs, a condition in which the optic nerve becomes less effective. At this point, messages are unable to get through from the eyeball to the part of the brain where sight is formed. RP affects both eyes and is a degenerative change of the retina. Most people with RP are registered blind or partially sighted because of their inability to see in the dark, with the visual field slowly decreasing in size, even in a good light (see Figure 8).

*Albinism*

In this inherited condition, the pigment layer which underlies the retina is absent from birth, and may be linked to lack of pigment in the skin and irises. Albinos often complain of photophobia, that

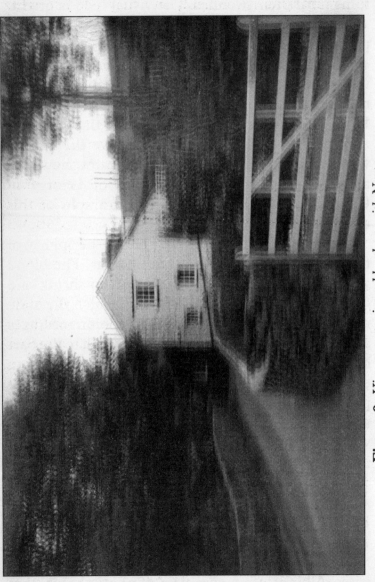

**Figure 9:** *View as experienced by those with Nystagmus.*

is, an intolerance to light, and may need to wear tinted glasses.

## Nystagmus

This is an uncontrolled wobbling of the eyes, which may be linked to infantile cataract, or albinism. In most cases, though, it is not possible to define a cause. The involuntary movement of the eyes makes it difficult for sufferers to see detail clearly. Sufferers often adopt unusual head posi-tions in an attempt to tighten up the muscles that move the eyes, thus reducing the unwanted move-ments to a minimum (see Figure 9).

## Glaucoma

Mostly found in people over the age of 40, glau-coma may rarely affect infants and children. Pressure increases within the eye if aqueous humour is over-produced, or is prevented from being channelled back into the bloodstream. High pressure damages the nerve cells at the head of the optic nerve where they leave the eye, by not allowing oxygen to perfuse out of the small blood vessels in the optic nerve head. Peripheral vision is affected first, and then central vision; if not treated at an early stage, some sufferers will lose their sight entirely. Occasionally pain may occur, but this is a rare symptom, most cases being detected as part of a routine eye examination.

\*   \*   \*

All these conditions may qualify the sufferer to be registered as partially sighted or blind, but the situation is rarely that simple, because one condition is often intruded upon by another. For example, Retinitis Pigmentosa extinguishes the peripheral sight, leaving a slowly diminishing central vision, but the person may be already short-sighted with cataracts forming. (See George's case, Chapter 3.) There may also be flashing lights from PVD. Overlapping conditions are fairly common.

Yet a person registered blind seldom loses the ability to see light and dark and may continue to have just sufficient sight to enable them to get around a familiar place, such as their home, to attend to their personal needs and even, with a little help, to live alone. There are aids and gadgets which help towards independence, although the 80% of information which is received through sight can never be totally replaced.

## Very Rare Conditions

*Akinotopsia*
There are other very rare and unusual conditions, one of which prevents the person from seeing any movement whatsoever. In such a case, tea coming out of the spout of the teapot and into a cup resembles a golden glass tube. The only way of knowing the cup is full, without the use of a liquid leveller, is

to put the fingers in the saucer and feel the spilt tea. Consequently, a person with this condition would be in extreme danger out on the street, as traffic cannot be seen to be moving: it is at point A and then at point B.

Fortunately, this terrible condition is extremely rare, and is one into which research is being carried out.

*Hysterical Blindness: Julia's Story*
The strangest condition I have encountered, however, is hysterical blindness, as demonstrated by Julia's story.

Julia had fallen down the steps at a London Underground station. Badly concussed, she was taken to hospital, where she remained for several days before regaining consciousness. When she began to recover, she was convinced that she was totally blind. She could, in fact, see, but her brain was telling her that she was unable to do so.

When I met her in her own home, Julia had been fully cane trained and used the long white cane when out in the street. She had also adopted a rather rolling gait sometimes seen in other blind people when they are walking. We sat down to talk, during which time she laughed at a kitten playing in a far corner of the room. She later began to show me pictures in a catalogue and we discussed the items she was pointing out, and she was convinced she was totally unable to see. Fortunately this is a

very rare condition, but one that is extremely difficult to live with.

## Dreams

Blind people dream, just like and just as much as
the rest of us. It is said by psychiatrists that
without dreams we would find it very difficult to
live our daily lives, as in dreaming we often find
solutions to our everyday problems. Although it
is very difficult to find totally blind people who
have never experienced the sight of images to
explain how they dream – as those who lose their
sight in later life are able to – we know they
dream and have similar experiences, although not
in picture form.

*Eileen's Story*
A single woman now in her mid seventies, Eileen
has been blind from birth. She is an excellent
Braille reader and loves reading. When I asked her
what it was like to dream, she was rather puzzled
and had difficulty in explaining to me how she
recognises her dreaming. Finally, she said, 'Well,
you know when I'm reading how I live in another
place with the characters in the book – that's what
dreaming is, really.' Eileen has no perception of
images or space or colour, but her dreams are full
of feeling, not just touching and feeling with her
hands, but her reactions to sounds, conversation

and situations to which she has an emotional reaction such as fear, or joy.

Most people who have been sighted still dream in colour, even though they have lost the ability to see colour in their waking life. Few people without any sight, who once had sight, however, dream of faces, yet they are aware of people in their dreams and seem to know their identity. It is quite common for people who have been severely visually impaired for a long time to dream of themselves in situations where they know they are adult and yet all the images are much larger than life, as if they were still children. Trees are enormous, walks take forever, shops and buildings are gigantic, as they would have been to a small child and whilst they loom large, they seldom appear to present a threat. Many people who have once been able to see appear to enjoy their dreams, although of course when they are troubled the dreams become distorted, as with everyone else.

### Joyce's Story
Joyce is now 80, but she remains a dignified, lady-like and thoughtful person. Her sight began to deteriorate after she lost her husband some ten years ago and now she sees very little. In common with many other blind people, she dreads being taken out for a meal, whether it is in a public place or in someone else's home. Her

anxiety is so strong that it provokes very bad dreaming. Dreams of her own shameful behaviour, which include other forms of this besides spilling food, create further anxiety in her waking life.

Dreams engendered by fears of public disgrace and humiliation are quite common with blind people, but inconsistencies of time, place and feelings are nonetheless very pervasive. These dreams are all in colour, sometimes of real and sometimes of bizarre situations, where many people are present but unidentified – the only identifiable person is oneself, exposed and disgraced.

### Celia's Story

Celia feels that her dreams take place somewhere in the City of London, where she used to work. She suddenly comes upon a dress shop where all the windows are full of beautiful pink evening gowns, all of different materials and styles. This is a vivid, repeated dream, although Celia cannot account for it in any way. Some blind people, like Celia, get pleasure from their dreams; others, like Joyce, find their anxiety heightened.

### Stanley's Story

Stanley was in the Royal Navy during the war. Although he is no longer able to see very much, he constantly dreams of being on board ship and watching mountainous seas.

## Hallucinations

There is, however, a phenomenon experienced by approximately 40% of blind and partially sighted men, women and children, of all ages, which is known as the Charles Bonnet Syndrome, or CBS. It takes the form of hallucinations which are always three dimensional. Charles Bonnet was an eye doctor practising in Switzerland in the middle of the eighteenth century. Bonnet was so concerned about his patients who suffered this phenomenon that he wrote a paper about it; as he was the first to recognise it, the condition now bears his name.

Since then, very little attention has been paid to this sometimes very unpleasant syndrome. In 1989, researchers found that a mere 46 cases had been recorded since Bonnet's writing in 1760. At last it is now being taken seriously and researched, particularly by Dutch, American and some English ophthalmic researchers.

The condition varies from person to person and appears to have no common origin. The images seen may be pleasant or very frightening and embrace everything a person might see throughout their life. It could be a vase of flowers or a bowl of fruit sitting on a table, but only the table is really there. Or perhaps you might see a wonderful view of a lovely garden or pastoral scene. Or looking out of your window on to an average suburban garden you might have, instead, a view of the sea with yachts and seagulls – but no sound. There may be ugly faces and menacing people lurching towards you. Most people are emotionally affected, with some experiencing fear, whilst in others a great sense of pleasure is found.

## Grace's Story

Now in a residential home, Grace asked to see me on a day when she was feeling a bit lonely. She is a 79-year-old widow with a caring, loving family and is totally blind. There is no question of her being able to see, as she had her eyes removed some time ago. All at once she startled me by saying, 'Oh look at that.' When I asked her what she could see, she said, 'I didn't know we were on a bus route here. Oh, and I have just seen that bus, look at it, it's at the bus stop.'

Anxious to know more, I asked her what was happening and she told me that people were getting on and off the bus and those who got off were walking away. Grace was so excited that I sat quietly until she said, 'Oh, what a pity, it's just driven off! Well that was wonderful, I haven't seen anything like that for so long and I had no idea that buses came right past here.' Her home is nowhere near the buses and Grace was facing a completely blank wall. Despite the fact that Grace had heard no sound, she had enjoyed the experience.

*Clara's Story*

Not so for Clara, who is a grandmother originally from the north of England. In her eighties, Clara is a lovely, gentle, sweet woman whose daughter-in-law suggested she might come to see me. I found her to be rather depressed and very anxious. Her hands, which she placed in mine to give her the courage to speak, were shaking and her fingers were constantly moving. We talked about her incurable eye condition, for which she had been registered blind for about two years. I learned that she had been widowed some years before losing her sight and, although their life had been very hard, she missed her dear husband very much.

Clara appeared to be very well balanced and certainly not hysterical, but her anxiety was almost palpable. I guessed what might be the problem, hoping to hear it from Clara's own lips, until about ten minutes before the session was due to close when I asked her, 'Are you seeing things?' She burst into tears. She told me that she had been seeing gruesome faces for a long time, they frightened her and she feared she was losing her mind. She wept profusely, partly with relief that she had been able to voice this awful condition. I tried hard to be reassuring and told her that it was not psychological, and that many people shared it with her. Clara had tried to tell her doctor, who prescribed a sedative and advised her not to talk about it.

I then suggested that we might have weekly interviews for a little while to see if we could find out any more about these frightening faces. When she described the apparition, it seemed to be very like the face of Punch in the Punch and Judy show and eventually I asked her if she had ever had a holiday when she was a child. She said no, but she went on Sunday School outings and so we tried to remember what she had seen at a northern seaside town many years ago. She named a number of things and eventually came to the Punch and Judy man and stopped. 'That's what I am seeing,' she said, 'Punch.'

Talking and reassurance helped Clara to come to terms with what she was seeing and although she was always frightened, she saw the apparition less frequently. I was delighted when she had no further need to come and see me, as the apparitions appeared less often and she felt she could go and live with her daughter-in-law again. She was feeling well and having a good night's sleep at last.

No one has ever come to any conclusion about these hallucinations, yet few are willing to talk about them for fear they are losing their mind. Sighted people and many doctors treat it as imagination, but there is nothing psychotic about this condition. There are no sedatives with which it can be treated and unless the person is given the opportunity to talk about it openly, it can have disastrous effects. The fact that it does not seem to happen to people who are born without sight may be the clue to its cause. It may be discovered eventually that the optic nerve carries images to the brain in a distorted form, even when the eyes are no longer working properly, if at all, in the same way as a phantom limb is felt after its amputation.

## Ursula's Story

Not everyone has Clara's ability to ignore something so unpleasant. This is so with Ursula, who had a very serious retinal condition, but managed to live alone in a warden-controlled flat. The first time she saw grinning, bald-headed men lurching towards her with their arms outstretched, she screamed and collapsed on her kitchen floor, where she was found by the warden, who called her doctor. He prescribed some medication and indicated to the warden that it might be a mental condition. Ursula gave up her flat and is now in a residential home, where there is always a carer on duty who can be with her should this hallucination recur.

## Hilda's Story

In Hilda's case, the apparition seems to be sparked off by colour. Hilda suffers from cataracts with a right hemianopia. She manages well with the little sight available to her, but recently the white standard rose tree in her garden, which was in full bloom, was replaced by a lady in a white dress. At about the same time, when she went into her sitting room, there were young men and women sitting on the settee, all dressed in the same colour as the settee, or the carpet. Their lips appeared to be moving as if they were speaking to one another, but as always there was no sound. Occasionally they seemed to split up into more of the same sort of people and walk about the room looking at things, always in total silence. This happened in other parts of the house, but only where the carpet was the same colour as the carpet in the sitting room; these people have never appeared in any part of Hilda's house which does not have that carpet or furniture. She now laughs and tells me that she goes to the settee and sits on them and tells them to clear off. 'They don't go,' she says with a smile, 'even though I am sitting on top of them.'

*Betty's Story*
There is one form of this condition, however, which is extremely rare and when it occurs seems only to affect visually impaired women over the age of 65. Betty, a highly intelligent retired teacher and intellectual who enjoys music and the arts, is in this category. In this case, there is nothing to be seen, but that which invades her life was felt in the form of crustaceans which she could feel crawling over her. Unfortunately the people she told about this gave it no credibility, dismissing it out of hand. The

need then to talk about it to someone who would believe her became urgent and I agreed to see her. Betty is very articulate and described these 'creatures', as she called them, in considerable detail.

We arranged to meet for sessions on a regular basis, during which time Betty described what had been happening since I last saw her. These visits continued for almost a year, during which time the tortuous and terrifying creatures appeared less often and were replaced by furry animals who were friendly and companionable. When she is more relaxed and sitting comfortably, one Betty calls Drowsy Cat will jump on to her lap and a kitten will creep into the crook of her arm. The most extraordinary one of all is one she calls Spider Monkey, which rides on her back with its tail hanging down and its arms around her neck. She feels this even when she's shopping, as well as when at home. There is no fear with these 'furry friends' and Betty now feels more distressed when they are not present than she does when they are.

I understand that several cases of this kind have been reported to medical organisations and the phenomenon is now being researched.

Some people who have been born without sight will never see anything at all. It is important for them to learn to live in their own world of darkness by being properly educated and cared for. Thus enabled, they will have the confidence to live full and satisfactory lives in a community where they are valued. None of the phenomena which I have highlighted in this chapter is likely to affect them. The long list of things which blind people see, encompassing the distortions from flashing lights to all types of hallucinations, are experienced only by those who were born into the world of sight and later go into a world of blindness. There they almost always see something, even if it is only the difference between daylight and darkness.

# 3

# *Barriers*

The barriers that are experienced by the blind and partially sighted are both physical and emotional. In this chapter, I am going to look at both of these areas.

## Physical Barriers

The shut level-crossing gates, the 'no right turn' sign, the 'closed' notice on shop or office door, are some of the barriers that sometimes prevent us all from doing what we had planned to. Others occur in the form of rules and bye-laws which are there for the common good, but which may prove irksome: no smoking, keep off the grass, no pets allowed.

People in wheelchairs are, of necessity, much more aware of, and hampered by, physical barriers that prevent their access to public buildings, libraries, cinemas, polling stations; being barred by steep roadside kerbs, steps, narrow doorways and lack of lifts. Efforts are now being made, through public awareness and legislation, to put these things right.

For those with little or no sight, physical barriers include busy roads, the crossing of which constitutes a stressful experience, even with a guide dog or human help. The presence on pavements of signposts and other street furniture, placed there by private enterprise or by a local authority (and perhaps shifted if roadworks are taking place), is also hazardous. Sometimes street signs have projections at face level; the blind person with a white cane may locate the post but not the dangerous extension overhead. Trees at the sides of urban pavements may cause hazards for those who are visually impaired. Yet when such trees have to be removed, the contractors may not take into account those for whom their work could pose a risk.

One victim in this area was Edna, who fell into an unprotected hole left when a tree had been removed, in a road she knew well; the workmen had left without erecting the required protecting barrier. The outcome of the accident was serious permanent pain and disability.

## Access to Information

Not having access to information is a barrier that active, independent blind and partially sighted people tend to find the most frustrating. A quick survey of the means whereby sighted people can acquire information – from books, newspapers,

pamphlets, directories, dictionaries, encyclo-
paedias, letters, computers, television, radio and
telephone – shows that only in the last two are
blind people more or less on a level footing with
the sighted. (See Chapter 1: Communication, in
the section on Alternative Means of Communication, for details on access for the blind to
print and other media.)

## Being 'Taken Over'

Sometimes with the best of intentions, other
people – family, friends, helpers – erect barriers of
frustration that are the reverse of helpful.

*Joanna's Story*
As Joanna's sight was failing, in her very tidy
kitchen she rearranged some items for her own
convenience. Her family, however, could not
accept that things were not as symmetrically placed
as they used to be, that the tea now was kept in a
distinctively shaped tin labelled 'sugar' ('As if that
matters to me! *I* know where it is'). Their regular
shifting of her kitchen's contents, she said, was
driving her demented.

*Lucy's Story*
Lucy needed to buy a birthday card for a teenage
boy. The cost was unimportant to her – she simply
wanted a humorous card. Her companion,

however, took her from shop to shop, rejecting this one as 'too expensive' and that one as 'not nice' or 'a bit rude'. There was no chance for Lucy to say, 'But that's just what I want – to make him laugh!' The card finally bought was not at all what she had had in mind.

### Geraldine's Story

Geraldine's family were reluctant to accept her invitation to come for a meal, protesting, 'It's too much for you.' When they accepted, they would not allow her to complete the preparations, which she is quite able to do, but took over in the kitchen – leaving her alone in her sitting room. She found this hurtful.

## The Struggle for Independence

A man or woman who experiences sight loss in later life, and can still cope with independent living, knows that there are some very ordinary situations where they cannot manage without help. Examples of barriers to freedom of action and movement include serving food to guests, going to the bathroom in someone else's house, walking across an open space in the garden, small sewing repair or DIY jobs, wasting long minutes feeling around on the floor for the dropped coin or button, losing the house keys. Embarrassment is a constant fact of life – as, for example, when realising that the voice you have heard addressing someone in the crowd has actually been speaking to you!

Many older blind people are much saddened because their life-long habit of attending church services no longer provides pleasure, support or a sense of belonging, since they cannot read the words in order to join in the hymn singing. Instead, their sense of exclusion is emphasised by being obliged to stand silent while others sing.

### In the Street

Independence of movement outside the home for a blind person entails concentration, and very likely the counting of paces. Any interruption in the process – by a chance meeting, say – may result in the blind person's arrival not at the end of the road as planned, but into someone's garden or garage!

### In the Office

When a blind person is employed in an office, there is an absolute requirement on the part of the personnel officer to explain to other employees that the problem is sight loss, not 'learning difficulties'. This may seem obvious, but it must have been some such misconception that produced the circumstance where Louise, sitting at her switch-board, could hear a lengthy conversation just outside her open door between a manager and a director of the company. They were discussing in detail the highly confidential matter of methods they planned to use to 'get rid of' a member of staff. On another occasion, a manager told Louise that a group of Chinese people would be coming to visit the building, and asked her, in careful, slow speech, 'Do you know what a Chinaman is?' (Louise at the time was working for an Open University degree.)

Memos circulate throughout any ordinary office day, but experience shows that often they are not read to a blind employee as they appear, but only days later – if at all. Clearly this does not promote overall efficiency in the office, and it also shows a lack of thoughtfulness on the part of colleagues.

## Loss of Eye Contact as a Barrier to Understanding

*In a Social Context*

It is loss of eye contact – the importance of which has been dealt with in Chapter 1: Communication, in particular – which bars blind people from taking the initiative in a social context and obliges them to remain passive, often pre-judged and misunderstood. Take, for instance, joining an evening class for pleasure. Eye contact between members of the group will, from first meeting, lead to relationships being formed. Unless someone is sensitive to the blind person's failure to react in a 'normal' way, and is prepared to take the initiative, the blind person will continue to be excluded and isolated:

unaware of questions addressed to them by the tutor and discouraged from joining in discussions.

*Interviews and Assessments*
Another area in which lack of eye contact is a serious problem is where we are assessed by others, which takes place throughout our lives. Teachers, prospective employers, bank managers, insurance people, mortgage lenders, members of the medical profession and many others, make judgements about us and decisions that affect us. In this process, lack of eye contact is an enormous barrier – firstly to real communication and then to the development of self-confidence and independent worth. Unless interviewers and assessors are trained to be aware of what loss of eye contact means to blind people, they may not respond appropriately, and this barrier will remain in place. More seriously, assumptions will have been made in the course of these interviews which, unverified, can damage the blind person's prospects or well-being.

## Assumptions and Attitudes

I will now consider in more detail the sorts of assumptions constantly made about people suffering from sight loss, and the consequences of those assumptions.

A blind woman was buying a flat. She was entirely

competent to manage her own life and live there on her own, but other occupants of the building heard of her intention and raised so many objections born of their fears and prejudices ('She could very easily burn the place down!') that she was forced to withdraw.

A local survey which I made several years ago left no doubt that the most feared disability among able-bodied people is blindness, which they imagine to be total darkness. Maybe it is because we feared the dark so much as children that as adults we are reluctant to talk about it, or face it. Blindness is one of the last taboo subjects; fully-sighted people avoid it, create barriers within conversation and in their minds use myths and old wives' tales as a comfortable way of dealing with it. For example, it is strongly believed that when sight is lost the other senses all improve, but in fact one's other senses do not improve at all: if they appear to do so, it is only because they are being used more effectively.

Another assumption, that all blind people read Braille, is nonsense. Very few people indeed are able to read Braille fluently, and these are mostly those who were taught when they were children. But the greatest misconception is that when you are registered blind you have no sight at all. This is the cruellest mistake.

How do we interpret the term 'blindness' in relation to those who are registered blind and yet can see? The answer is that they have a residue of useful vision, even though it may be severely distorted (see Chapter 2: The Eye and What Blind People See, for further details on this). These people are probably the most mis-understood of all the visually impaired. They often feel embarrassed, because whilst carrying a long white cane, wearing dark glasses or even using a guide dog, they may still be able to read small print.

*George's Story*
An example of this was George, who had a little sight, just in the centre with no peripheral vision. In other words, he could not see anything around him, and when he was looking straight ahead he was totally unaware of where he was treading. He used a long white cane and, as sunlight was painful to him, on a bright day he always wore very dark glasses with side pieces to cut out the glare. One day he had to go on a long train journey alone. A porter took him to the train and found him a seat.

George did not want to spend the journey doing nothing; he could not see anything clearly through the window, nor read a book, because when he reached the end of a line of print he had difficulty in finding the beginning of the next line, so small was his field of vision. So he had equipped himself with the *Daily Telegraph* crossword, which he could manage as each clue was only a few words long.

The carriage filled up, and the train moved off. After a time, however, George heard mutterings among the other passengers and became aware of a hostile atmosphere. He realised that they were drawing conclusions about him, assuming that if he could manage the crossword then he could see: he was not blind, he was a cheat.

George put away the crossword and waited miserably for the journey to end. He had to ask if he had reached his destination since he could not see the name of the station. He told me that as he fumbled his way to the door, feeling for the steps with his cane, he was very thankful to find his brother there to meet him.

## Josie's Story

Another example in a completely different setting happened to Josie, an apprehensive elderly lady in a large hospital ward. She had very little sight indeed. A hospital employee came and sat on her bed and accused her, 'You're an old fraud, aren't you!' She was deeply shocked and could not imagine what she had done, till the explanation came, 'When I waved my hand in front of your face you flinched. You could see it! You're not blind at all.'

That sort of behaviour is unforgivable, but it happens because so few people understand the effects of blindness, and make cruel assumptions, in this case about an unassuming and vulnerable lady.

Similar misunderstandings arise in other situations, for example, in a big store where a blind woman is buying clothes, whether accompanied or on her own. She asks for a mirror, and the sales person at once makes assumptions about the customer's sight. In fact, the colours she sees may be distorted, patterns on the material invisible, and only a small portion of the garment visible at one time. But for all that, a mirror may provide some useful information to a person struggling to use to the full what sight remains. In some large stores, company policy has led to more training being given by professionals to staff, so that they can better understand the needs of blind and other disabled people.

I hope that the issues discussed in this chapter may lead to a heightened awareness on the part of all who meet blind people, whether casually, socially or professionally, of what their problems and needs are and how some of the barriers they encounter in their daily lives can be removed.

# 4

# *Hazards and How to Avoid Them*

Simple everyday things may become dangerous monsters to those who are newly visually impaired. They not only have to learn new social and daily living skills, but also how to make themselves recognised by other people. This chapter aims to show how with a little forethought and willingness, many potential accidents can be avoided.

## The Quest for Independence

The chief aim of most visually impaired people is to retain or recover their independence, to which end mobility must be the key. But everything which has to be learned in this new world of darkness or distortion increases the struggle to re-establish a purposeful and self-sufficient life. This is very stressful and at first adds to the burden which sight loss has already created.

It needs to be borne in mind that orientation (knowing your exact location in space) is the key to mobility, just as mobility is the key to independence. The two principal tools which have been adopted for teaching independence to blind people are the long white cane and the guide dog. Learning to use the cane comes first.

*Mobility Training*

In mobility training, the fullest possible use is made of the remaining senses of hearing, touch and smell, and also of memory, sense of direction and any residual vision. A professional, experienced mobility officer will tailor a programme for each student, to ensure the minimum amount of stress, knowing that patience – together with perseverance on the part of the student – will bring great rewards.

Even people with another disability besides blindness may benefit considerably from some parts of the training. For example, elderly folk too frail to use a long white cane or a dog can often learn to orientate themselves within their own home and to improve their daily living skills. Likewise, timid and nervous people may eventually gain the confidence to walk down the pavement outside their own house without holding on to someone else. The mobility officer will give due consideration to a student's medical condition (many drugs can cause drowsiness and lack of concentration, and greater care must be taken with someone who is diabetic).

The course of instruction will usually begin by teaching efficient methods of travelling with a sighted guide and finding safe ways of negotiating steps and stairs, doorways, getting on and off various forms of transport and moving through narrow spaces. When confidence has been established between the guide and the visually impaired person, early training with the cane will begin, usually indoors at first. Then things will progress until train and bus travel, various road crossings and tactile mats may be used by the individual with confidence, all the while developing the other senses to the fullest degree possible.

This training will inevitably improve all the daily living skills at the same time. Until mobility training has been completed, however, the Guide Dogs for the Blind Association will not consider further training in the use of a guide dog, though this may be the blind person's ultimate goal.

We owe a debt of gratitude to those who devise these training schemes and to the dedicated people who teach them to blind people in our society today. But the society in which we live is growing, becoming faster and creating more and more hazards. Therefore, it is supremely important for mobility training to be available whenever required, and for fully sighted people to understand some of the particular problems encountered by blind people as they seek to acquire mobility.

## Some Major Hazards

*Doors*

The ordinary door is a potential hazard when it is neither fully opened nor closed. When ajar, its edge can be easily missed, even if the blind person's hand is slightly extended protectively. A severe blow can be sustained to the side of the head and can even damage the eye. All doors can be dangerous if taken for granted, such as the revolving doors and lift doors in public buildings and cupboard doors in our homes. Most especially, doors on all forms of transport: for example, doors which have to be slammed on older railway carriages; doors which automatically open and close, as on underground trains; doors on motor cars when the driver is in a hurry or fails to heed your request for help are all potential sources of danger for those unable to see.

People are sometimes taught to find the top of the open car door, and then the seat with the other hand. But an even better method is to ask to have the left hand located on the edge of the car roof above the door space, while the right hand locates first the back of the seat, and then the seat itself. Then, keeping the hand on the roof, you can turn, sit on the seat and swing your legs into the car before releasing the left hand. This method prevents an accidental knocking of the head. It is

important not to put the hand on the pillar
between the two doors if you are getting into the
back of the car – the front door can all too easily be
slammed on your hand, which is acutely painful
and often permanently damaging.

## Stairs and Steps

Staircases within the home need to be protected at
the top by a barrier at bannister-rail level, attached
by hinges at one side, swinging easily open as you
ascend the staircase but closing firmly against the
other side to prevent an accidental fall. Worn stair-
carpets can cause accidents and need to be
replaced or repaired promptly.

Still more dangerous to the unwary than indoor
staircases are concrete or stone steps such as those
leading down to underground stations. Frank, on
his way to a concert in an unfamiliar church hall,
where the entrance was some seven steps above
ground level, was unaware as he walked in that he
was barely an inch away from a flight of stone steps
going down to his left. He had missed them with
his cane and would almost certainly have fallen
down them but for someone who noticed and
grabbed his arm. He no longer goes to concerts
alone! People with no peripheral vision are particularly vulnerable in such situations.

A fall of this nature could well cause greater
injury to a blind than to a sighted person. It is
seldom realised that when any of us falls, at the

moment of loss of balance, the body engages through sight to protect itself as far as possible from the eventual impact. In other words, we can see whether we are falling a few inches or a few yards. But if we cannot see, the impact of the fall may be far greater. Impact fractures do not always come at the point where the limb hits the ground: the impact of a hand on the ground during a fall may cause a fracture between elbow and shoulder, rather than in the hand or wrist, and the long-term damage may be more severe.

## Obstacles in the Street

These are a danger to everyone, but especially when sight is poor. Such obstacles include: overhanging branches; untrimmed hedges; cars parked on the pavement; children's toys and bicycles lying wherever they were dropped; advertisements on metal stands outside shops and cafes; and roadworks involving electric cables, scaffolding and pieces of machinery. A trained cane or dog user will ultimately be able to negotiate most of these, and busy roads are less terrifying once the technique of traffic assessment has been mastered, particularly when the locality is familiar. Knowing when and how to seek sighted help rather than venture alone is of paramount importance.

## In the Garden

By contrast, the garden may seem a less hazardous

environment, but here too are dangers for those whose sight is impaired. Bend over a bush or plant to enjoy the scent, and the supporting stake could seriously injure the face, or worse, the eye. It is very easy to become disorientated on, say, quite a small lawn, or elsewhere, if a handrail has not been installed. Windows which open outwards on the ground floor can also present a danger, and all garden tools should be used with great caution.

## In the Kitchen

It is essential for the blind person to know precisely what cleaning materials they are using. Some are more dangerous than others and it is important they are easily recognised. It is sometimes asked whether one method of cooking is safer than another for a blind person living alone. Both gas and electricity present hazards, and it is easier to stick with what is familiar. A microwave oven is probably the safest cooking method, and those who learn to cope with a simple model may progress to a computerised, talking microwave!

The method of cooking used is largely a question of choice – and budget. However, whatever it is, it should be remembered that grilling food is difficult without sight (it tends to burn); pans on top of the cooker boil dry unless attended to; chip pans containing hot oil are lethal; frying is always hazardous; all electrical equipment should be switched off when not in use; and that sharp knives, especially, should be treated with great respect.

In preparing even a simple meal for one, clear away as you go, keeping everything tidy and in its own place. Simplicity is the watchword; recipes can be put on tape; jars and cans labelled in Braille; cookers and washing machines can be fitted with marked dials; scales can be either talking or with weights. With practice, many blind people can and do manage to look after themselves quite satisfactorily and safely.

Visually impaired people sometimes find themselves in an institution such as a hospital, residential home or a day centre, where they may be eating and drinking. In such places, other people sometimes fail to realise how unpleasant it can be to put your hand on a sticky surface when you cannot identify the substance. It may be only jam or spilt tea which has not been cleaned up, but the instant reaction is 'ugh!' and the imagination may work overtime! It is really important, for the sake of blind people who have to feel their way everywhere, that the surfaces they have to touch are kept clean.

*Electric Sockets*
Most electric points are still to be found low down, just above the skirting board. A blind person must use two hands to locate the socket and the holes in it, so all the points should have a built-in safety

factor. A further problem is that often the points are below a shelf or table from which the blind person risks a blow to the back of the head when rising, with possible further sight loss.

## Fires

Fires represent a particularly dangerous hazard, whether bonfires in the garden, coal fires in the grate, free-standing electric or other fires. It must be made impossible for anyone to fall onto any of these. Smoking constitutes a special fire hazard, particularly when the person who lights the cigarette cannot see very well, lives alone and easily falls asleep. It should go without saying that no visually impaired person should ever need to light a bonfire.

## Noise

Although thought of as a nuisance rather than a hazard, noise may be just this when it blots out sounds that are needed to replace information no longer available through sight. At a function where everyone is talking at once, someone without sight can become completely disorientated; very loud music can produce a feeling of total isolation; the roar of traffic on a busy road can cause great anxiety, as no other aural information can be picked up.

This is all due to the fact that 80% of one's intake of information comes naturally via the eyes; it is never possible to compensate adequately by using other senses, and when the second most valuable sense – hearing – is also blocked by excessive noise, the ability of that person to be in touch with him or herself is taken away, causing much distress and loss of confidence. Even for blind people well trained in mobility and able to travel alone, a busy railway station, for example, is a stressful place.

## Guiding the Blind

Most sighted people are confident that they would be capable of taking a blind person across a road. But without a little instruction, this is seldom the case. People usually respond to a request for such help by taking the arm of the blind person and either dragging or pushing them, often gripping the arm like a tourniquet! Sometimes instructions are shouted, to add to the discomfort. I was once 'helped' on to a bus by a well-meaning lady who, as the bus drew up, gave me a push in the small of my back, saying 'There you are, on you get!' – without telling me exactly where I should step. As a result, my tights were torn, my shins bleeding and I felt very 'un-helped'!

Even in hospitals, staff may not know the right way to guide a blind person. Queenie was pulled and hurried down a long corridor, tripping because of the speed of transit, while the nurse repeated 'Come along, come along, we are used to people like you here!'

The correct and safest method of guiding a blind person is in fact the easiest of all: the blind person is asked to hold the top of the guide's arm, with the palm of the hand on the inside of the arm and the thumb on the outside. The guide's arm is kept close to the chest, so the hand is on a level with the guide's ribs. No pressure is needed – a light touch by the blind person will be sufficient to feel exactly where they are going. This method can be used in any situation, even when walking through woodland where there are no paths, or going shopping in a large store, or anywhere inside a building.

The only information required is when you are going to turn left or right and, when coming to steps, whether they go up or down. On steps it is often better, should the blind person wish it, to put their hand on the handrail and let them go up or down on their own. (The guide should ask if they prefer this, not presume to decide for them.) Guiding is a very short-term commitment and it really needs great care and concentration to take someone from A to B. It may seem obvious, but the guide should not abandon the blind person en route or go off to talk to someone else.

When going through doors, the guide should open the door and help the person being guided to go through in front of them, closing the door behind them. When showing a blind person where to sit, put their hand on the back of the chair (or, if faced with an armchair, on the arm) and help them to locate the seat. I was once 'shown' to a theatre seat, only to discover that it was at the end of a row, with no outer arm rest, and that I had sat myself sideways with the stage on my left and my legs in the aisle.

'Guiding' must never mean telling a blind person to go across a busy road. This happened to Timothy, who was taken off the kerb and instructed to 'Hurry up, there's just time to get across'! Fortunately he had the sense to step back and find someone else to guide him across. This sort of dangerously inadequate 'help' is almost unbelievable, but it happens through ignorance and lack of imagination rather than deliberate unkindness.

All living involves risks and hazards, specially for those who lack sight. With determination, these people can achieve a high degree of independence, though they will always need help at some points from the sighted. More and more people are coming to realise the value of this interdependence and how much society owes to all who show determination and courage in overcoming major disabilities.

## Warnings to the Sighted

Well-intentioned sighted people may cause confusion, distress or even serious risk to a blind person who is in the process of negotiating a staircase or other tricky passage (with or without the help of a guide dog) and especially while going *down* stairs or steps. A blind person has to concentrate single-mindedly during any such manoeuvre and it is unsafe to divert their attention or interrupt the rapport between the working dog and its owner, unless really necessary. It is wise to leave any accosting for social reasons until a point of safety has been reached.

A word of warning also to dog owners who allow their pets to roam off the lead: care is needed to ensure that a working guide dog is not distracted – or worse attacked – by any free-ranging dogs.

# 5

# 'To See Ourselves as Others See Us'

When an individual suffers sight loss, their close family, relations and friends are often also thrown into a state of emotional chaos, in which their own fears of blindness may be projected on to the person who is now visually impaired. In this state of mind, and without knowledge or experience of this condition, they may only be able to imagine what their *own* needs might be, should the situations be reversed. Rather than asking outright how they could help, they become anxious and over-protective.

For this reason, the help offered may be the opposite of that required, but with understanding, patience and a positive attitude – plus a sense of humour – family life may be improved for all concerned. It would be unwise, however, to expect this level of care from strangers who have had no experience of helping the blind, but do what they can – give directions, cross a road or chat on bus journeys. We are very grateful and could not manage without them, but sometimes their intervention or chance remarks require a sense of humour . . .

## Out and About

*'Us Human Beings . . .'*

I was out with a group of friends who were all using white canes. It had been snowing and as the snow had filled the gutters, it was difficult for us to find the edge of the kerb. The road was wide and rather busy, with an island in the middle, so it must have been obvious that we were in trouble when a lady came up and asked if we needed some assistance. We accepted her offer with enthusiasm and she shepherded us to the centre island in safety. Here we had to wait for a while before continuing to cross the other half of the road. While we were waiting there, she suddenly realised why we had been in difficulty in the first place and said, 'I've never thought about this before, but the snow to you people must be just like the fog to us human beings.'

We did manage to get to the other side of the road, where we thanked her profusely and parted from her before falling about with laughter. None of us had ever supposed that when you lose your sight you opt out of the human race altogether. On reaching our destination we did wonder, rather cynically perhaps, if this gave us an even greater freedom than those who could see.

## 'Don't They Dress 'Em Nice'

The assumptions which people make may often give rise to laughter and here I think back to the time when I was at the rehabilitation centre in Torquay. It was early summer and three of us decided to go into the town to a little cafe for a cup of coffee. As the town sea front was crowded with holiday makers, two of us decided to walk together while our friend followed just behind. We had all learned to use the cane and we two, walking in step with our canes swinging in unison, were thoroughly enjoying the fresh air and the freedom. We went into the cafe, sat down and ordered a coffee.

A few moments later, the friend we were waiting for stumbled into the doorway almost doubled up with laughter and speechless. It seems that remarks made by people as they passed us walking in the opposite direction were overheard by her. The best such remark came from a lady who said to her companion, 'Don't they dress 'em nice up there.' We decided that we must all have better dress sense than we had previously given ourselves credit for!

## 'I Can't Cross the Road Till the Aeroplane Has Gone'

It is often the unexpected which causes a disbelieving laugh or a wry smile. I was once waiting to cross a busy road and must have seemed to be waiting an unnecessarily long time, because a passer-by came up to me and asked, 'Are you waiting to cross the road, or to meet someone?'

My answer was, 'I'm waiting to cross.'

The reply came, 'Well you can go now, it's quite clear.' But I explained I would not be able to cross the road until the aeroplane overhead had completely passed. This brought a disbelieving laugh and I tried to explain that because it was obscuring the traffic noise, until it had gone I could not be quite sure there was nothing coming.

The woman just said, 'Oh, I see', and walked away, failing, I think, to understand that safety depends upon noise not being obscured by drills and aeroplanes and things.

### 'The Wrong Sort of Box'

A few years ago, there was a shoe shop in our local high street which sold exactly the kind of shoes I liked and, in need of a new pair, I went into the shop. Somehow, though, it didn't feel quite right and I wondered if the shop had changed hands and nobody had told me. There was none of that lovely smell of new leather.

Before I could say anything, a lady came up and quietly asked how she could help me. I started to tell her what I needed and she began to giggle. When she had recovered, she simply said to me, 'I'm awfully sorry my dear, our boxes are much too big to contain shoes.' At that point I realised what was wrong. I was in the undertaker's next door! She was extremely kind and it was good to know that we could share the joke together.

## A Case of Mistaken Identity

On another occasion, my daughter took me to buy some clothes. I knew exactly what I wanted and the assistant brought things which I felt were not suitable, although I couldn't see them. Someone was telling me with absolute certainty that these things would suit me and they would look very nice. With coldness, I said quite firmly, 'Please do not try to persuade me, they are not what I have come here for at all.' I was sure it was one of the other assistants trying to sell me something that I was not prepared to buy.

As I finished making my point, politely and clearly, a familiar hand caught mine, as a voice I now recognised said, 'All right Mum, you don't have to talk to me like that, I was only trying to help.' It had not been another assistant talking to me, but my poor daughter, whose voice had been badly affected by a rapidly deteriorating sore throat. On this occasion it was I who had made an assumption which could have been very hurtful – when you are unable to see, not only do you have to learn to laugh at yourself, but also to be careful what you say.

*Learning to Laugh at Ourselves*
Despite these examples, no one should imagine that all the *faux pas*, misunderstandings and assumptions which cause such mirth come from sighted people – blind people themselves make many more. Learning to laugh at yourself when you feel foolish or embarrassed, and to look happy when you are feeling wretched, is an art which has to be learned in order to survive.

I was once told by an acquaintance that she felt blind people must be the happiest folk in the world. 'They never look downcast,' she told me. I was at a loss, unable to reply for a moment or two and then with what I hope was a smile, I simply said, 'I'm afraid we can't afford to be anything else.' Once the visually impaired have learned how to laugh at themselves, then it is acceptable for others to laugh with them: it takes the sting out of a mistake.

*Party-Going*
So, what about the invitation to a party being held in a neighbour's house when all the other neighbours are invited as well? It's good to know that even though you are blind they want you to be part of the whole gathering, but it is with trepidation that you accept the invitation and are reminded that if you can get there, someone will see you home. The day comes, the moment arrives, you hear the music as you are knocking at the door. You are made so welcome.

Many people are already there in the large room where the furniture has been rearranged. You have to be taken to the chair where you are going to sit for the rest of the evening, usually at the far end of the room. There are a few people sitting there already to whom you are introduced – perhaps an aunt who would love to have someone to talk to because she is in plaster from her hips to her shoulders; and an elderly gentleman who is hard of hearing and finds conversation difficult. You do your level best to communicate with them both, but with no eye contact and their disabilities, it is very hard.

The wine and food are brought to you and your host comes over from time to time, sure that you too are having a wonderful evening. Most of the other guests, however, are standing in the middle of the room talking to one another, a few may be dancing, while you just long to be going home.

At most of these get-togethers, the 'elderly and the infirm' find themselves in a corner of the room which is away from whatever is going on, on the assumption that any one person with a disability will automatically have some sort of empathy with another.

Many people who suffer sight loss in later life feel isolated and no longer part of their own social group. More often than not, these occasions only serve to reinforce that empty feeling of loneliness. Most blind people, particularly those who have no partner, are pleased to be included in such a gathering – hoping this one will be better than the last – but learning that it seldom is.

*Hurting Unintentionally*
It is, however, very easy, when blind yourself, to forget that there are occasions when the people who are with you are also blind, especially when you may have recently lost your own sight. This situation occurred recently when a married couple, both blind from childhood, entertained a blind friend who had been able to see until a few years previously.

The evening went very well and just before she left, the friend made a light-hearted remark to the husband, which would have been recognised as a joke by any of her sighted friends, but at which the wife took umbrage. Where her sighted friends could have seen the body language and the smile, the blind couple were unable to, causing a cooling of what had been a very warm friendship. If this incident were related to other sighted people, it would probably cause astonishment that such innocent fun could be so misunderstood as to cause someone to feel hurt.

## Eating Out

The social niceties are very difficult to carry out when you are unable to see what you are doing.

There are many people who would love to go out for a meal, but become so frightened of embarrassing someone else, that they never accept an invitation. This usually only affects people who have once been able to see.

Even going to a pub for a sandwich lunch is enough to terrify some people. Whatever sandwiches they order usually arrive cut into four little triangles covered with a finely chopped salad, making them very difficult to find and pick up with the fingers. Often the filling is so exotic as to be likely to fall into your lap before you get it to your mouth. It takes a lot of practice and experience to negotiate these things, especially for older people, given that sandwiches were not often served in that manner until a few years ago.

When dining away from home, it is sensible to take a well-laundered table napkin with you, whether you are a man or a woman. It takes courage to tuck it into the collar with other people sitting around, but it gives a great deal of confidence and people soon get used to seeing it. It is much better to do that than to spend the rest of the time with a messy tie or a spoilt dress.

In these situations, it is also a good idea to ask what is being put on your plate and where it is. I am reminded here of a talk I gave to some young children in a junior school. They were fascinated when I suggested you could put the food on someone's plate and tell them, as if the plate were the face of a clock, that the meat was at 6, the potatoes at 12, the cabbage at 9 and the carrots at 3.

Later, the children all wrote a little composition which they were allowed to read onto a tape and send to me. I was delighted to read it; they had listened well and some of the things they wrote were very interesting, especially little George's, 'Mrs Daniels told us how to turn a plate into a clock – you put your meat at 6, your potatoes at 12, your cabbage at 9 and the carrots at 3. Then Mrs Daniels knows what the time is.' He knew exactly what he meant.

## Eating with the Family

Sadly, though, there are occasions when an apparent lack of good table manners can cause a great deal of unhappiness. Marjorie was a woman in her seventies who had lost her husband very suddenly. The shock caused the onset of a serious eye condition, which led to total blindness. Her daughter was unhappy about Marjorie living at home alone and she and her husband suggested that she move in with them. Marjorie ate with the family, but because she was unused to being blind, she frankly forgot sometimes and instead of asking to have things passed to her (feeling that she was being a nuisance) she would put her hand to where she thought they were, often knocking something over or touching some food unintentionally.

A crisis occurred during one breakfast when her son-in-law could bear it no longer. Marjorie had reached out for the cruet and put her hand straight into the marmalade dish, having already found the butter by putting her fingers into it. Marjorie burst into tears and the son-in-law left the table. Marjorie knew that this could not be allowed to go on. She did not mean to do anything wrong, but it was upsetting to all of them. She decided to go and live in a residential home. This was difficult for her to do, but it was even harder to accept that a person like herself, who had always paid attention to good table manners, could cause her daughter so much unhappiness.

## 'What Am I Wearing?'

A blind person's forgetfulness may also be the source of a little embarrassment and a lot of laughter!

*Eileen's Story*
Eileen had been taken by her daughter to buy some clothes and was now the proud possessor of a new lightweight jacket. The following week she was going to an old girls' reunion and one of her school-friends was going to bring her home. When she arrived at the hall, her new jacket was hung up in the cloakroom and, reunited with her old friend, the two of them had a very happy evening.

Time passed and some people began to go home.

Eileen then described the jacket to her friend, who went to the cloakroom to look for it. She was gone for some time and returned to say there was no such jacket to be seen. They waited until everyone had gone, only to find that a jacket of similar style, but not the same colour, had been left behind. They decided that someone had mistakenly taken the wrong garment and would be sure to return it. Feeling very uncomfortable, Eileen wore it home. Her son answered the door and the friend stepped in quickly and apologised for bringing his mother home in the wrong coat.

The son, however, said, 'No she hasn't, she is wearing her own jacket.'

'No,' said the mother, 'the one I bought was a beige colour with a striped red and yellow lining. This one is blue, isn't it?'

Her son's answer was, 'That's the one you wore when you left,' and everyone began to feel a little uncomfortable.

'I'll telephone my daughter,' said mother.

Her daughter then reminded her that there had been two jackets. 'I know you liked the beige one,' she said, 'but it didn't fit you as well as the blue one, which was the one you finally bought.'

Mum had a very red face. When you cannot see, you do sometimes forget what colour something is, but you do not expect loss of memory to cause such embarrassment or such amusement.

### 'Dressing in the Dark'

It is true to say that everyone in the world makes mistakes, but sometimes blind people make mistakes that have to be seen to be believed. Anyone who has had to get dressed in the dark knows how carefully clothes have to be selected. On one occasion, I had to leave very early to get to my destination in time for a meeting, so I set my clothes out the evening before, but not my shoes. At the last minute, and in a rush in case I missed my transport, I took my shoes out of the cupboard, flung on my coat, harnessed my dog and we were away.

It was not until I was on my way home in the early evening that I realised I was wearing one black and one navy blue shoe, similar in design, but obviously different. At first I was embarrassed, then angry that no one had pointed it out to me during the day. Eventually I decided that if anybody had said anything to me I could have laughed and said, 'I have another pair just like these at home.'

## Mistakes in the Kitchen

Culinary difficulties arise where people who have recently become visually impaired continue to prepare meals and do the cooking. More than one apple pie has been taken out of the freezer and served up with vegetables and gravy . . . And it is impossible to describe what a casserole tasted like when a can of raspberries went into it instead of tomatoes!

*Helena's Story*

The prince of all culinary errors was made by Helena, who invited her son and his new wife for Sunday lunch. She was very careful with the first two courses, keeping them plain and simple, and it all went off quite well, but the *piece de resistance* was to be a Pavlova. The base turned out beautifully, the cream whipped nicely and the strawberries were all ready. Just before it was assembled however, she thought what a marvellous idea it would be to stir in a few raspberries, which were in a little bag in the top of the freezer.

Helena was so thrilled she had managed it better than she imagined, until it came to serving. Her son asked, 'What are these bits of green in it, mother?'

With a sinking heart, she realised that the packet of raspberries which she had picked up was a packet of chopped green peppers. Of course it was possible to pick out the bits of pepper, but Helena felt dreadful, having tried so hard. Her efforts were spoiled because she had not checked things carefully enough. I believe it is now a family joke that she will never be allowed to live down.

## Towards Independence

Being visually impaired means you have to wait for someone to find the time to help you do the simplest task, which you would have done in a moment when you could see – altering the boiler clock, sewing on a button or reading a letter. It is very hard to have to ask someone who is kind and willing to give up their own time to do these small, but necessary, tasks.

Being unable to read, at the shops or the post office you are never sure whether you are in the right place or ought to have waited at a different counter. Blind people who are trying to run their own homes find that a good part of every day consists of waiting. But as one young housewife said to me, 'I couldn't do what I do if I didn't have to wait such a lot, because it gives me time to plan tomorrow's meals, the weekend shopping, and many other things' – real positive thinking!

## Being Taken Advantage Of

Most blind people find that travelling involves a lot of waiting. Even if you hire a car, *it* may arrive late, but *you* have to be ready on the dot. Waiting at bus stops is worse; bus services in towns are often unreliable and it can take two hours to do a twenty-minute journey.

Moreover, it is extraordinary how many people think they have the right to ask you the most personal questions while you are waiting at the bus stop in a queue – how and when you lost your sight, whether you can see anything, how you manage. No other disabled person would be accosted like this and it is very difficult to prevent yourself from getting into deeper conversation or from being rude. Occasionally, with questions such as, 'What's it like, love?' 'Is it all dark?' 'Would you like to feel my face and see what I look like?' a polite 'No' does not really satisfy.

It was, however, on a bus that I first discovered there are some people who will take advantage of those who cannot see. The bus was packed. I sat on the last seat just inside the door behind the driver with my guide dog at my feet and my holdall on my knees. The person next to me was as close as it was possible for two people to be and it was a difficult situation. My holdall was open at the top, as I had been shopping, but I was holding the two handles firmly together.

I was suddenly aware of something moving, and putting a hand into my bag I was shocked to find another hand there. It was quickly withdrawn and I asked what on earth the woman was doing. She said she thought it was her bag, even though it was on *my* knees! She did not even apologise. I felt very shaken that someone would take advantage of me in that way. And many years later, I employed someone in my home, only to discover that I had been grossly overcharged and exploited and my trust betrayed. The woman was, of course, dismissed, but it is a very hard lesson to learn that when you are unable to see, you have to be careful whom you trust at all times.

## 'Blind People Are Not Really There'

It is strange how people will often talk in front of someone who can't see, as if they had made the assumption that unsighted people are not really there. A blind member of staff, for example, has no eye contact with the other employees, and sub-consciously becomes invisible to them. It may be exciting to hear something no one else knows, but it puts a tremendous burden of responsibility and confidentiality on to the person who has overheard a conversation that should be private.

## No Magic Wand – Yet!

The sight of someone walking with a cane can have a strange effect upon some people. Once it was my turn to be open-mouthed with disbelief. I was trav-elling by bus, using the long cane, and as I got up to get off at the end of my journey, a youngish gentleman got out with me and offered to take me across the road. As it was a busy main road, I was glad of his help. He asked which way I was going and walked along with me. There was something he wanted to ask. I had no objection and so we continued together.

The man was trying to pluck up the courage to put a question to me, and so I deliberately slowed down to give him the opportunity. He wanted to know what the cane did. I explained that in itself it did nothing, it was the way I used it and what I interpreted from its use which helped me to find my way.

'Oh,' he said, 'I thought it was some wonderful device which when you held it, enabled you to see.' There are some strange myths and stories which sighted people believe, but that is perhaps the strangest one I have heard. Let us hope that one day a magic wand really will be invented which, when it is held, will enable blind people to see!

## Christmas, Grief and Gifts

Christmas is a particularly hard time for so many of the lonely blind people I see in the course of my work. They cannot bear to go to church, even though they have been used to going regularly. They can no longer read the carol sheets or follow the service and it holds no meaning for them any more. An invitation to someone else's house, though accepted, is dreaded, for they sit and wait to have their Christmas cards read to them, which often means waiting till everyone else has read theirs. What seems like hours later, it is possible to have their own gifts unwrapped and described to them, with the name of the giver. Quite often, much of this information becomes mixed up – that is, if they have to rely on their memory in order to thank people.

The giving of gifts to those who are unable to see often presents a problem to their sighted friends and relations and themselves. Just imagine sitting in a room, where you have been for the day, when someone approaches to give you something. You are handed a parcel and expected to be delighted with the gift, even when you don't actually know what it is. A lack of response, or an apparently negative one, can cause offence so easily to the giver, who completely misunderstands the situation the blind person is in.

As for what gift to give a blind person, chocolates are a great favourite. One of my clients told me she had six boxes in her refrigerator after last Christmas – and she doesn't eat chocolates very often. Flowers are another favourite, but if you are unable to arrange them or to see when they are dead, they are likely to give more pain than pleasure – although the thought is always appreciated.

Many of the blind women living alone whom I see tell me they just wish their sighted friends would give them some *time*. 'It would be wonderful,' I am told, 'if someone would sew a button on for me, or take me to a shop where I could choose something for myself.' Younger blind people, of course, are caught up with their own age group and are much more dynamic and positive, knowing well which records they want, for example, and what they want to wear.

Older people, unless there is something they specifically need to have replaced, appreciate those gifts which are going to help them in a more personal way, yet may have no knowledge of what the big stores have to offer. Fortunately, the RNIB and other organisations (see Chapter 9 for details) have a great range of games and other gifts for people of all ages, for friends and families of the visually impaired who wish to give something a bit special.

The stories which I have quoted in this chapter show some ways in which visual impairment leads to diminished social abilities, and the consequent loss of many of one's former joys and pleasures. They illustrate too how loss of sight is perceived, or misunderstood, in the world around it, and in particular the degree to which relationships with friends and acquaintances – and most of all with one's family – are affected and even distorted.

# 6

# Blindness in Old Age

According to a survey conducted by the RNIB in the late 1980s, at that time there were approximately one million people in Great Britain who could be registered as blind or partially sighted; a further million were very near eligibility for registration. (Registration is voluntary, though it has to be authorised by a consultant ophthalmologist, so the figures are not precise.) The survey showed that as least 75% of these people were over the age of 60, and with increasing numbers living to 85 and beyond, it is evident that blindness is likely to be a matter of growing concern in our society. This chapter will mainly deal with those past retirement age.

## Approaching Old Age

The process of ageing is a natural phenomenon to which every living thing, including the human animal, has to adjust. Heredity and environment, upbringing and experience, are the influences through which the individual learns to deal –

usually more or less adequately – with each stage in life, and in particular with the limitations and frustrations met as old age approaches. The sort of person we become depends to a considerable extent on the sort of person we have learned to be in earlier years. Thus, the man or woman who has developed positive attitudes to the changes and chances of life may face even the onset of blindness with courage, and with a firm resolve to remain independent for as long as possible.

Of course, health factors also play a part in determining quality of life and will need to be considered. But one experience is common to all of us as we grow older – that of loss: loss of peer group, of relationships, of status, often coupled with an overwhelming sense of diminishment, which makes us resist change and cling to the familiar. Such experiences of loss, which occur quite rapidly to some of us in later years and which may include gradual or sudden loss of sight, are a form of bereavement, and need to be understood as such.

The frailty of many elderly people is due to the slackening of tendons, muscle wastage and, in particular, poor circulation, which means that the brain receives insufficient oxygen, owing to inadequate blood supplies. Short-term memory loss is very common, as is a deterioration in hearing. (Where the latter occurs to those who are visually impaired, an important warning must be given to carers: because hearing aids often give a distorted sound, which may seem to be coming from the wrong direction, it is unwise to tell a blind person using a hearing aid to 'come here' across an intervening space.)

Other signs of ageing may be corrosion and wearing away of the joints, bowing of the back and gnarled and twisted hands and feet, making the person feel small and distorted. Hence feelings of impotence arise as the world appears bigger and people in it more threatening.

## Libby's Story

This is exemplified by one ageing blind woman, Libby, whose future was being discussed and determined by a 'conference' of carers, social workers and relatives, at which she was present. Having no eye contact with those making decisions for her, and no possibility of reading their body language, she felt herself being reduced to a state of uncharacteristic passivity and helplessness as she listened to them making plans for her removal to more secure accommodation 'for her own good'.

These plans were subsequently carried out, riding rough-shod over Libby's feelings and wishes. She afterwards spoke of the passive submission with which she had found herself reacting, prevented by her blindness from intervening on her own behalf.

*Ida's Story*

Ida, in her late seventies and blind, lived alone in a
ground-floor maisonette, which she had agreed to
move into in order to be near her son. Each day she
was visited three times by carers who got her up,
got her meals ready, and put her to bed. Relatives
would drop in every day to keep an eye on her, and
she had an alarm bell for emergencies at night.

The pain in Ida's eyes could be alleviated only
by steroid drugs, which caused her weight to
increase, so walking was difficult. With little to
occupy her mind, she slept a good deal during the
daytime, so those who visited her presumed that
her mental state had deteriorated, which was
certainly not the case.

When I first met Ida, it was difficult to draw her
out, because for so long no one had really tried to
engage her in conversation. But gradually, in the
course of a number of meetings, she began to
reveal some of the events of her active and fasci-
nating life. It was a chance mention of audio books
which proved the key to unlocking her past. What
was all too clear to me was that although her physical needs had been well catered for, Ida had not
been encouraged to talk about herself and there
was no mental stimulus for her once lively,
educated mind. Over the weeks I saw a total trans-
formation of her personality: she became 'alive'
once more.

The moral of this story is self-evident: Ida had at

least five people who visited her daily, but no one to talk to . . .

The feelings of impotence exemplified in the two case histories above may also be projected outside oneself, on to other people and the world in general. A very common everyday instance of this could be, 'The food they give us isn't grown as it used to be, and when they get it, they don't know how to cook it.' The complaints may be justified – though the sense of taste does diminish with age – but some element of paranoia may cloud our minds as we advance in age and become less competent in ourselves. It is easier to put the blame 'out there' than to admit to our own failing powers. It is all the more understandable in those whose vision is impaired, when facts cannot be verified by sight, as, in our example, the food on the plate can not be seen.

We all have aspects of ourselves that we recognise but keep in check under a social veneer. With age, the defences crumble, revealing hidden traits of greed, childishness, dominance, inferiority or even sadism, which can no longer be completely controlled. Elderly people who lose their sight may sometimes be seen to step into this phase of old age more easily than most because, by retreating into their new world of sightlessness, they lose touch with the day-to-day world. They therefore find it difficult – and maybe even unnecessary – to hold on to these defences. Abandoning the defences may bring release, because the categories of 'should' and 'ought' have been relinquished. In this self-accorded absolution from guilt, some quite mischievous satisfactions may emerge, that compensate for the loss of powers previously enjoyed.

In this phase, the elderly blind may easily become fretful and demanding, expecting too much of their now middle-aged children, who often bear the whole responsibility for their care, and understandably feel resentful, in some instances even resorting to neglect or bullying. Here is a situation where counselling may be urgently needed, in order that both carers and cared-for may retain their dignity. Reciprocity and mutual respect come only when each values the other in equal measure. Otherwise, carer and cared-for alike may regress into childish – even infantile – behaviour.

Some people do experience in old age a new sense of freedom to be themselves, caring less about social conventions or the opinions of others. Such release may, however, be harder for the elderly blind, because their disability has brought them into a world of distortions and often darkness. There they continue to be beset by the turbulent feelings – alternatively negative and positive – experienced by all who lose their sight. They are likely to need support to preserve their integrity, and some will profit from professional counselling. This may be true whether they are living independently or in a residential home.

## Residential Care

It is to this latter group, in residential homes, that I now turn.

*Making the Move*

However obvious the need and desirability of such a move, the fact remains that giving up independent living, home surroundings and the possessions of a lifetime, perhaps losing the companionship of a pet, constitute a major trauma. It takes only a little imagination to realise that for someone who has lost their sight, this renunciation and removal from familiar surroundings can entail additional stress and distress.

How often it happens that, perhaps with the best of intentions – 'We're seeing to it all, mother, you have nothing to worry about' – the house is sold, furnishings are shared out or given to a charity. Those greatly valued possessions – ornaments, perhaps old photographs, or the offerings made at school by the children – have been classed as 'rubbish' and thrown away. As if these treasures were any less precious because the blind person can no longer see them! Yet this person feels the need to be grateful, not to hurt *their* feelings – they have been so kind! – while all the time it feels as though the pattern of daily life, and the blind person with it, has been wiped away.

In the residential home, bodily needs are attended to, but the purpose for living and the well-known landmarks have gone, with consequent disorientation and confusion. Some of the bigger charities run specialist homes for the elderly blind, where conditions are, on the whole, very much better than in larger homes or geriatric institutions where blindness is seldom understood.

## In Residence

Most visually impaired people in residential homes have been bereaved by the loss of a spouse, or other close relative, and often the sight loss is due to the shock of their bereavement. Their world is a lonely one. In residences where old people can see one another, even if they are unable to move about, they can catch someone's eye, call out to them and have a conversation – or a row. But with no eye contact it is very difficult for one blind person in a roomful of blind people to engage in any exchange. Only the person in the next chair, within touching distance, can be reached, and that person may be asleep or unwilling to respond.

It may be that a resident has a real wish to communicate, to express opinions, views on life, on politics, religion or other controversial topics. Carers should encourage any sort of communication or expression of ideas, even if by today's criteria they appear out-of-date. Some of the better homes provide residents with mental stimulus, such as simple entertainments, games, or organised discussions. Such activities are of great value.

Some residents do find that the change has been to their liking, and appreciate the comfortable room, regular meals, presence of other people and little things to do. When I asked Ted, a blind ex-serviceman now in a residential home, what advantages he found in being old, he said with enthusiasm, 'I don't have to worry any more. My nephew sees to my pension and the tax man. If I'm not well I get taken to the hospital in a car; when I get there I'm put in a wheelchair and all the doctors and nurses are nice to me. Then I come back to the home where I'm warm and comfortable, and there is somebody here to look after me again.' After a pause, however, he added, 'I just wish my Audrey were here to share it with me.'

Some have likened being in a residential home to 'being on holiday' and another, very unhappy at first, became reconciled after a spell in hospital and spoke appreciatively about 'coming home'.

## Caring with Understanding

In relating to and caring for those whose lives have spanned most of the twentieth century and the beginning of the twenty-first, it is important for counsellor and carer to appreciate the enormous changes through which these people have lived, and to be able to get alongside them with a working knowledge of social history. Without it, young people enter the caring professions with the best of intentions, but ill-equipped to understand where old people 'come from', what, in their present outlook, is due to childhood influences, their religious upbringing, the effects on them of two world wars, or the hardships of the depression years of the 1920s and 1930s.

As an example, take Neil, 93 when I met him, blind and in a residential home. In his early years he enjoyed the benefits of money and position, being a naval officer by profession. Later he managed large estates in South Africa. Whilst Neil appreciated the care he received in the home where he was ending his days, he greatly missed his wider horizons and the companionship of the kind of people with whom he had spent most of his life.

Those who care for the elderly blind, whether living alone in their own home, with a relative, in sheltered accommodation or in residential care, can help to make their lives less isolated by a sympathetic realisation of the ways in which things have changed in their lifetime. Changes in the fields of science and medicine, for example, and moral and social attitudes, have brought about a climate far removed from the norms by which elderly people have lived since their early years. Much that today's world takes for granted will need explanation. Allowance must be made, and respect paid to beliefs that have served the elderly well through their lives, even if society today has largely discarded them.

The psychologist Eric Rayner calls old people the 'living historians of our society'. Those who care for, or counsel them need to respect them in this role.

# 7

# *Blind People in Need of Medical Care*

Sickness does not discriminate, and blind people are not immune to the accidents or illnesses which may strike any of us. When this happens, we may pay an initial visit to a doctor's surgery and need medication, perhaps self-administered. More serious illness could involve a spell in bed, perhaps with some nursing care. Or the GP may suggest a visit to a hospital, to see a consultant, for tests or outpatient treatment. Surgery may be needed, resulting in a spell as an inpatient in a hospital ward. In all of these circumstances, treating a blind patient requires more forethought and care than may be immediately apparent.

## At the Surgery

Let's begin with a blind person's visit to their GP's surgery. The staff will most likely be very helpful, probably knowing in advance the patient and their needs. Likewise, most doctors are considerate and make patients feel at ease. Blind patients, however, need to be given a little extra reassurance. Before even the simplest procedures, they need a preparatory word, 'I am going to feel your shoulder,' or 'Let's try moving that ankle.' This may seem obvious, but it does not always happen.

## At the Pharmacy

The doctor frequently hands over a prescription which has to be taken to, and later collected from, a pharmacy. The chemist's shop may be busy, but vital precautions need to be carried out to ensure that the prescribed drugs and the dosage can be distinguished and taken correctly. For example, if ear-drops and eye-drops are in identical containers, they are easily confused: ear-drops put in the eyes can at best cause pain, at worst damage. Similarly, tablets should be in differently shaped or sized bottles (once-a-day in a smaller bottle, twice-a-day in a larger one). Gargles and liquid medicine may be easily distinguished by a sighted person, but feel identical to someone unable to see; the bottles should be different in shape or texture.

The shop assistant must also check the patient's name and address so as not to hand over the wrong medicine. I have known this to happen, and when it leads to someone being rushed into hospital, as one of my clients was, there is little comfort in hearing, 'I'm sorry'. But given thoughtful aid in these ways, most blind people can manage, even when they live alone.

## Home Nursing

Should the blind patient be ill in bed at home with the district nurse visiting the house, it is important for the nurse (or any other helper) to remember that words such as 'this' and 'that' or 'here' and 'there' are meaningless to someone unable to see what is being indicated. Some patients, particularly the elderly, become disorientated even when in their own home. This is usually because the patient is under enormous stress. Eighty per cent of normal information intake is through sight, and there is little compensation through the other senses, so already the patient is more stressed than sighted people would be. Any illness will increase this stress-load considerably, even if the patient is resting in bed.

## Outpatients

In the case of a hospital visit, many blind people who are mobile (that is, with a long white cane or a guide dog) may prefer to go alone. They might, however, find unexpected difficulties on arrival. To begin with, they cannot read any of the written directions which are to be found in corridors and waiting areas, above doors and so on. Neither can they catch anyone's eye in order to ask for directions, so help is needed from the moment they arrive. It is good to be able to report that some Accident and Emergency departments are better organised these days than formerly; they have a reception nurse on duty at the entrance who will make sure that the right procedures are adopted, finding help when necessary.

Unfortunately, experience shows that other areas of a hospital may not cater so efficiently for a patient without sight.

*Lionel's Story*

Lionel had an appointment in the eye unit of one of the large London hospitals. He sat waiting for four hours before anyone came to help him. When he finally reached the consultant's room, he was told that they thought he had not arrived. The unfamiliar place, the lack of anyone to help, coupled with an urgent need to go to the toilet, made the long ordeal particularly nerve-racking. Whilst it is usually better for a blind person to be accompanied on hospital visits, it is not always possible, and in Lionel's case it was not thought to be necessary; his appointment was, after all, in an eye unit . . .

## Going into Hospital

When a visually impaired person becomes an in-patient for any reason, the care and understanding offered by hospital staff will help that person's recovery significantly, maybe even shortening their stay. Fear of the unknown and unfamiliar is felt by most people who go into hospital for major treatment – an anxiety state which is greatly heightened when the patient is visually impaired. Most of the help needed is simply verbal explanation: being told where you are; who you are speaking to and their role or status; what is going to be, or has already been, done; where things are; and the function of any medical equipment which may need to be attached to you.

These are not the only ways of helping someone who is unable to see. An interview with a lady whose blind mother had been in two different hospitals was very revealing. It is instructive to look at this case in detail.

*Ethel's Story*
In her sixties, widowed and with two married daughters, Ethel was taken into a local hospital to have gallstones removed. Blind with glaucoma which had been considered untreatable in her earlier years, Ethel was a good person, having been

brought up to be polite and not to give trouble to anyone – particularly to those in authority – and she assumed that in hospital she would be properly looked after.

In the first hospital, this was the case; with her agreement, they wisely put a notice above Ethel's bed, stating in bold capitals that she was blind. As her daughter said to me, 'That was good: never did I have to say "Why don't they realise my mother is blind?"' Everyone entering the ward knew the lady in that bed was unable to see – visitors, nursing and cleaning staff, therapists, registrars, consultants – all of them were immediately aware of her problem.

During her three-week stay, Ethel was contented; every bit of treatment was explained to her, everyone spoke to her, ensuring that she took her drugs and ate her meals. They were careful to put her bed near to the door to the toilet, so that once she could get up she might be able to take herself safely there and back. Even though, as it turned out, she never managed this, it had been thought through as a possibility. She recovered relatively fast and her daughters took her home. From there she went into residential care.

Some time later, while in the home, Ethel had a bad fall, breaking her hip, and was sent to another hospital some distance away. The words I heard from her daughter this time were, 'It was really awful; they were unable to appreciate the need to

place a notice above her bed to say she was blind.'
As a consequence, poor Ethel had a terrible time.
In her five-week stay, there was nothing on the
ward to let anyone know of Ethel's disability.
Consequently, with changes of staff, it took a long
time before even some of the nurses realised that
Ethel was blind. When her family visited her, they
found themselves constantly having to inform or
remind hospital personnel that she could not see.

When visitors to other patients sometimes
spoke to her, Ethel was unable to respond as she
could not know it was to her they were speaking.
At other times someone might be talking to the
patient in the next bed and Ethel would answer,
feeling humiliated when she realised her mistake.
No one ever came and put their hand on her arm,
as would have been appropriate, saying, 'Hello
ducks, I've come to clean round your bed.' She
had no conversation with anyone. This alone
made her age terribly, and she became disorientated and distressed.

Occasionally, Ethel would be required to get out
of bed and sit in a chair, but not always on the same
side of her bed, with the result that she was never
sure where she was or where her possessions were.
No one helped her with the contents of her locker,
and because she was afraid of going to the wrong
locker, she could not find her clean clothes or other
things until a member of her family arrived to help.
Her bed table was constantly being moved – swung

round, pushed away to the foot of the bed, or simply not there at all. Her drinks were meant to be readily available as she was supposed to have a high fluid intake. However, because of the varying positions of her table, she was too afraid to try to locate them in case she knocked them over, and so she went for hours without drinking. Her warm and milky evening drink was put on her table without her being informed: no one ever ensured that she drank it while it was still warm. And in the night, her fear of knocking things over meant that Ethel did not drink at all.

Once, her daughter, arriving in the evening, found three little plastic medicine pots on Ethel's tray, two of which still contained capsules. She had no idea how long they had been there. A nurse was brought out from the office to find out what was going on. The capsules had been there for hours; the person who had put them there on each occasion had simply said, 'Here are your tablets Ethel,' and walked away, leaving her unable to know 'where' they were.

Ethel's condition deteriorated so much during her five weeks in hospital that when her daughters entered the ward, they would hear her quiet voice, like that of an old, old lady, repeating piteously, 'Please, help me; please, somebody help me!' All this distress could have been avoided so simply: a notice above her bed, such as she had had in the first hospital, would have informed everyone coming into the ward, in any capacity, of Ethel's disability, and enabled them to care for her appropriately.

## Mealtimes

Mealtimes can be a problem. As we saw in Ethel's case, not only was she unaware that food had been put on to her table, but when she was able to find it she had no idea what was on her plate. This situation is easily remedied by referring to the round plate as if it were a clock-face, with 6 o'clock nearest to the person, 12 o'clock furthest away, and 3 and 9 to either side. In this way you can describe easily how the items on the plate are arranged.

It helps if foods which may require cutting up are supplied already cut, and the tactful offer of a spoon to make locating and eating the food easier may be appreciated. It is also helpful to provide some means of protecting the person's clothing; paper serviettes are not much use, but a tea towel or a tabard could be supplied, or brought in by someone in the patient's family. Eating without spilling food is particularly difficult to achieve without sight at the best of times – it becomes a nightmare when you have to eat while still in bed and perhaps feeling unwell.

## The Effects of Light

It is often not realised that visually impaired people are affected – sometimes painfully – by the direction and quality of light. Thomas was confined to a hospital ward after an appendix operation. He had a retina condition which meant that his eyes were peculiarly sensitive to sunlight, and his bed was opposite two uncurtained south-facing windows. He felt 'trapped' and the pain in his eyes was excruciating. 'I felt as if two car headlights were bearing down on me.' On the other hand, Harry, who needed all the light he could get because his eye problem was within the lenses, found himself in a dark corner of the hospital ward, so unable to make use of the sight he possessed.

## Trapped in the Day Room

In the Day Room attached to most hospital wards, the television is usually on all day – a fact which may please many patients, but to those who are unable to see the screen, it can become a form of torture. Sighted people may believe that pro-grammes on TV can be followed without a person seeing the action, but this is usually not the case. For this reason, it would be much kinder to let a blind person sit out of bed and listen to the radio or their talking book through a headset, which would disturb nobody.

As illustrated in Chapter 1, however, there are people who are registered blind and yet can enjoy television: those who have no peripheral vision find that their world is reduced to the size of the small screen, and whilst they cannot walk about easily (bumping into things and losing their way) they find that sitting watching the screen is a great pleasure. Unfortunately, there are so many different ways in which sight becomes blurred and diminished that it is always wiser to ask whether the individual wants to 'watch' television.

## A Personal Nightmare

I once found myself stranded in a TV-dominated Day Room – part of my own hospital nightmare, which was all too real. I had to leave my hospital bed to have an angiogram, and to travel by minibus to the cardiac unit, which was in another building ten minutes' drive away. I had been told nothing about what my own doctor referred to as 'this test', whilst the hospital personnel, rather alarmingly, spoke of it as 'the operation'.

Because of pressure on the ambulance service, I had had to leave for a 1.00 pm appointment at 8.30 am, at short notice. So, clad only in night attire, I was rushed down in a wheelchair to the waiting transport. On our arrival at the other building, the driver found a wheelchair for me which had no footrest and only one armrest. He wheeled me as far as the open doorway of the Outpatients department, and abandoned me there. Two hours elapsed. It was late September and quite chilly. Outpatients came and went, presumably wearing outdoor clothes, while I sat there in my dressing gown and slippers, and began to feel cold. I must have been conspicuous – I heard people making remarks about me as I sat there – but only after an age of waiting did it occur to someone in authority that I should not have been there at all.

Then, after further delay, I was wheeled away, up to the top floor, through the female geriatric ward and into the Day Room where the television was on full blast. Somewhere along the route someone, despite my protests, whisked away my documents, which I had been told that morning to hang on to at all costs. I had no watch, no one spoke to me and I had no means of knowing who was there or what was going on. At last, I heard the one o'clock news announced on the TV – the time of my appointment in the cardiac unit! I shouted at the top of my voice, to attract someone's attention through the hubbub, for which I was rebuked, but eventually I managed to convince the nurse of my plight and of the urgent need for action.

Now everything seemed to be happening. A young porter was summoned with a fully functional wheelchair and we rushed through the ward, past the office where my documents were thrown into my lap as we sped past. Over half an hour late, we moved at breakneck speed along one corridor after another, into the lift, down several floors – a veritable fairground ride, but I was not even strapped in. The experience was alarming, and added to the terrible anxiety over what was about to be done to me. We arrived at last at the cardiac unit, where I was met by an anxious surgeon and his technical and nursing staff. They had presumed I must be somewhere in the building, but had been unable to locate me. They were obviously all most worried, since before an operation of this kind I should have been rested and given a pre-med injection.

As I was helped up on to the operating table, I remember feeling near to tears, though too exhausted even to cry, and utterly defeated. I knew even then that had I been able to see, I would have dealt altogether more positively with the whole humiliating situation. Now, however, everyone was kindness itself, and the operation duly went ahead. Afterwards, the surgeon ordered a proper ambulance, with a nurse in attendance, to take me back to the ward from which I had originally come, where I was made welcome with a cup of tea. I had the impression that everyone concerned was relieved that I had survived the ordeal, but no one was as relieved as myself!

## The Danger of Making Assumptions

It may be useful to clarify further why these traumatic experiences occurred. They happened because:

• For the convenience of the ambulance service, I was taken nearly five hours too early for my appointment

- To speed my progress from my bed to the minibus, at the driver's request, a wheelchair was used
- Therefore the driver assumed that I needed a wheelchair on arrival also – that I was unable to make my own way
- No one on or after my arrival looked at my documents or asked me any questions, so no one realised that I was blind
- All along, assumptions were made about me and not verified, and communication between departments in that part of the hospital was non-existent.

*Passing on Information*

In other hospital departments, the same sorts of non-communication occur. I have known cases where physiotherapists have spent time innocently instructing blind or partially sighted patients in the use of zimmer frames, which would be totally unsuitable – and indeed dangerous to use, for instance in a residential home. Both hands are needed to manipulate the frame, leaving the user with no means of knowing by touch where they are. Again, somewhere along the line, there has been a breakdown in the passing of necessary information between departments.

Communication between medical or nursing staff and their visually impaired patients also forms an essential part of their care. Hospitals, these days, are being modernised in the cause of efficiency, and although this may be achieved, sometimes this may be at the expense of these patients' privacy.

Sharon, who had recently undergone eye surgery, unfortunately without success, kept an appointment at her local hospital's ophthalmic unit, which has been modernised and is much more comfortable than formerly. But it is now almost 'open plan', with a series of alcoves for consultations, from where it is all too easy for those in the waiting area to hear some of what is being said.

Already aware that her blindness was incurable, while waiting to see the consultant Sharon could not help overhearing a doctor saying to another patient, loudly and with some irritation: 'Blindness! We don't talk about blindness here. We are here to talk about sight!' The remark might well have been useful and positive in its context, but Sharon, overhearing it and knowing she would never see again, was bitterly hurt, and broke down in tears once she was outside the hospital.

Sharon's case is one example of how modern hospital design fails to preserve confidentiality and the privacy of patients. Staff may not be aware how far their voices carry, nor realise the effect words spoken to one patient may have on another who is trying to cope with anxiety, stress or panic.

## The Need for Staff Training

We have seen enough examples of hurt and disarray caused to blind patients to realise that some basic staff training could greatly benefit patients such as these. Training of this nature is on offer through the RNIB and elsewhere, at a relatively small cost, to hospitals and other institutions, where specialist care is needed and its quality so important.

The consequences of not offering appropriate training to hospital staff are clear from the stories outlined earlier in this chapter. Staff in most hospitals and in other areas of residential care have little or no understanding of what it means to be blind. Much of what appears to be thoughtlessness is most likely due to the speed at which everything has to be done today. For example, one of my elderly clients complained that her cubicle curtains were not drawn while she was washing herself in bed – a fact she was not aware of until afterwards. Then she felt outraged: 'I lived through two world wars but this is the most humiliating thing that has ever happened to me,' she said. Another felt angry and rejected when she realised that the person she was talking to had walked away, leaving her to carry on the conversation 'into thin air'.

Older blind people may be particularly vulnerable if they go into hospital for the first time; they need to have hospital procedures carefully explained and be helped, for instance, to realise why a hospital gown, which they cannot see, has to be put on 'back to front'.

A particularly distressing case was that of one of my clients, Agnes, who went into hospital with a bronchial condition. She was allocated a bed in a dark corner of a large ward. None of the staff knew she was blind. She had no family nor visitors, and incoming staff did not know she was there. For 24 hours she had no attention, no food, no treatment, and being blind and very old she just lay there until she was discovered the next day, in a very distressed state.

My experience of running training sessions extends over the past 15 years, and includes working with nurses-in-training in teaching hospitals, the Postgraduate Medical Federation (with postgraduate dentists), BUPA nursing and residential homes, as well as trainee social workers, care staff, wardens of old people's flats and other similar paramedical groups. I have encountered enormous enthusiasm and gratitude from all those present and participating in these sessions. Sadly, however, because of changes in funding and administration, this area of training is no longer being authorised by management to anything like its former extent. Yet given that we live in an ageing society, where already 75% of blind people are over the age of 60, inevitably more visually impaired people will be coming into hospital. Some small additional outlay on staff training would lead to a very worthwhile meeting of their needs, lessening their anxieties and hastening their chances of recovery.

To illustrate what can be achieved, I am pleased to be able to mention one NHS hospital in Surrey which has received an unsolicited testimonial from an acquaintance of mine, whose elderly mother was recently admitted for a hip replacement. She is registered blind with a little residual vision; her lack of sight was recognised from the outset and catered for. Initially she was given a single room with a nurse assigned to her personally, and at no time was she allowed to become distressed. By the time she was moved to the main ward, all the staff knew of her visual impairment, and treated her with consideration. Needless to say, the sensitive nursing care she experienced in this hospital has contributed significantly to her recovery and her sense of well-being.

*Twelve Golden Rules*

In conclusion, I would suggest that the following Golden Rules, if adopted, would help to speed the recovery of blind patients and make their hospital stay a much less intimidating experience.

1. In general, words like 'here' or 'over there', or the pronouns 'this' and 'that', should be avoided.

2. At a first meeting, all health professionals and other personnel should tell the patient who they are and what their role is. The information should be repeated briefly on each encounter.

3. On admission to a ward, the patient should be told where they are. Their surroundings should be described to them and they should be enabled to feel the bed, locker and chair and get a sense of where these things are. Once the patient is familiar with their surroundings, their furniture should not be moved around without valid reason, and without informing the patient.

4. All hospital staff should know how to guide a blind person safely – without pushing or pulling. The blind person should always take the arm of the 'guider'. (See Chapter 4: Hazards and How to Avoid Them.)

5. Any technical equipment which the patient has to use, or will come into contact with, should be described and their functions explained. Similarly, all procedures to be undergone need to be explained.

6. The administering of any drug *must* be supervised, and the patient should know exactly where their required drink is. It should ideally be in a container that cannot be knocked over and spilt.

7. Staff approaching or leaving a patient should inform them – with a light touch – who they are,

why they have come, or that they are about to
go.

8. Ideally, food should be cut up and a spoon
offered, as well as a cloth to protect clothing.
The patient *must* be shown that the meal, or
drink, is within reach (exactly where) and told
what it consists of.

9. Cubicle curtains should be drawn to ensure
privacy: the blind patient can still be aware of
being visible at inappropriate moments.

10. All health workers must *believe* their blind
patients if they say that the presence of a
bright light, or lack of adequate light, is
causing them pain or difficulty. Adjustments
should be made to suit their eye condition.

11. A blind person wishing to listen to a book or
tape should not be herded willy-nilly into a
Day Room with a TV!

12. Finally, some means of indicating clearly over
a bed that the occupant is blind will be helpful
to all, including people visiting other patients.

# 8

# *The Value of Counselling*

During the early months of my training as a counsellor, I told a few acquaintances of my long-held determination to specialise in working with visually impaired people. Their reactions were largely dismissive, even though blindness was a field with which they were not unfamiliar. One response, 'Surely blind people do not require counselling', was discouragingly typical. I went ahead nevertheless, and very slowly the openings I had hoped to find began to appear.

Twenty years ago, counselling was much less readily available than it is today, and was far more limited in its scope. It was mainly concerned – in the public's awareness at least – with marriage guidance and bereavement. Some maintain that the pendulum has now swung too far and that 'expert' help is necessary for coping with any of life's emotional problems. I hope to demonstrate in this chapter, however, that the onset of blindness, be it sudden or gradual, causes such profound shock and presents such overwhelming feelings of loss, that even those with close friends or family support – and especially those without it – may require the skills of a trained counsellor. Indeed, as my experience narrated here will show, the families and friends may need help too.

The purpose of counselling in any sphere is to enable the client to voice and share their feelings of shock and grief in an understanding, accepting atmosphere, to enable them to come to terms with their traumatic experience, and so to 'pick up the pieces' of life and move on.

## Counselling for the Blind

When working with those who face sight loss, the counsellor needs to have a clear understanding of the variety of eye conditions and how they are caused (see Chapter 2). This knowledge enables the counsellor to gauge what the client is facing and how to appreciate any difficulties which may exacerbate the condition, even if these are not immediately expressed. In a word, to listen to what is *not* being said and respond to it. The result may be to release secret fears and anxieties in the client, as this example shows.

*Rose's Story*
I was asked to see Rose when she was living in a

residential home where she had been for approximately two years. Aged 80 and totally blind, she
was the mother of a large family with a number of
grandchildren. She had had a very hard life,
working until she became too frail to look after
herself, but had never been a moment's trouble to
any of the carers who were looking after her. This
changed, however, when she started complaining
about going to bed at night. Rose was quite sure
that she was being put to bed in a garden shed or
outhouse, where she was pestered by foxes. This
caused the staff to feel that she was losing her mind
and they asked me to see her. From what she told
me, I felt that she was probably hallucinating (see
Chapter 2).

I asked if there was any smell and if the foxes
made a noise.

Rose replied, 'Oh no, they just won't let me sleep
properly.' Once she had told me why she was afraid
to go to bed, I was able to explain to Rose that
seeing things when blind is not unusual, she was
not losing her mind and I would make this clear to
the staff who were worried about her condition.

## The Relevance of Bereavement Counselling

When counselling the visually impaired, the techniques employed in bereavement counselling are
often the most useful, as all loss can be felt as a

bereavement, including sight loss. The world they knew and loved with all its visual beauty has now been denied them for ever. This leads to a feeling of disbelief, an effort to open the eyes wider in an attempt to convince themselves that it is not really happening. These are not dissimilar to feelings we all have when someone near or dear to us has died. It is as if the sight loss is being mourned. Even the strongest person feels afraid and sometimes shakes physically with that fear. This may be accompanied by a desperate feeling that life will never be the same again and a depression which is over-whelming.

In general, bereavement counselling aims to enable the client to accept their life in its new form by accommodating the changes which have occurred, and then moving on. The four tasks involved in attaining this are:

- Accepting the reality of the loss
- Experiencing the pain of death
- Adjusting to the new environment
- Letting go of the old and taking hold of the new.

If we see sight loss as a bereavement, the appropri-ateness of these stages will be evident, and are illus-trated by the following case studies.

*Accepting the Reality of the Loss: Bruce's Story*
It is quite normal for someone who is suffering a

slow deterioration to do their best to hide the fact
from other people. Bruce was suffering from glau-
coma and was living alone. He alternated between
denial and shame and his mood swings took him
from self-pity to anger. Because of his denial,
Bruce would stand at a zebra crossing waiting for a
number of people to come to the kerb and then
join them as they crossed. In order to hide his
disability, he would make excuses for tripping over
something as he went along, or when he missed the
kerb. Even when he walked into a lamp post, he
would turn to a passer-by and say, 'Oh dear! I was
thinking of something else.'

During our sessions together, it became clear to
me that Bruce was using these evasive tactics
because he felt ashamed of losing his sight. I began
to feel that he would never accept his sight loss,
when fate intervened. His insistence on keeping his
symbol cane folded in his pocket resulted in a road
accident. At the following session, he still insisted
that his accident had been the motorist's fault, but
we both knew that this was not the case. The accident acted as the catalyst which enabled me, with a
little more encouragement, to persuade him to take
proper long cane training. Now, with his head held
high, Bruce is walking with pride.

*Experiencing the Pain: Shirley's Story*
In Shirley's case, sight loss was sudden and total.
Here denial was impossible, and therefore the pain

caused by the loss was overwhelming and acute. Shirley had to be moved quickly to a residential home and I met her very shortly afterwards while she was still in a state of shock. She had given up a beautiful home of her own because she was totally alone and had no one to care for her. Both her sight and her home were lost – a double bereavement.

Shirley felt numb, she was unable to think straight, she wept copiously and was severely depressed. She was experiencing the emotional pain of mourning, the expression of which was the focus of many counselling sessions. After we had worked through this stage with Shirley, she was suddenly taken into hospital for a short while. On her return, her first words to me were, 'It's lovely to be back home.' This was a real breakthrough and our frequent sessions since have enabled her to remain buoyant. She is now more positive and settled into her new environment.

*Adjusting to the New Environment: Andrew's Story*
Andrew's wife came to see me in desperation. Her husband had been diagnosed as having Retinitis Pigmentosa, and as a result he had had to take early retirement. He had always been active but was now in a state of depression, which I felt could become severe. He was reluctant to get up in the morning, sat in a chair all day, refused to do anything and was, 'Unlike the man I married', his wife told me.

I suggested she brought him to see me. We made an appointment and they arrived together. After the introductions, Andrew and I were left on our own. It soon became clear to me that his depression resulted from his inability to accept his sight loss. I also knew that it would be quite a long time before Andrew would lose his sight completely. The trust and rapport which developed between us over several months eventually enabled him to accept my suggestion that a guide dog could be a big help. Both Andrew and his wife became enthusiastic – the first time that such a feeling had been expressed by Andrew. With the new independence that owning a guide dog affords him, Andrew is now working part-time and enjoying life again.

Andrew's story exemplifies not only an adjustment to the new environment, but also letting go of the old life.

## Empathy

As every counsellor knows, certain strategies need to be employed within the counselling situation. The first of these is the initial joining or engaging with the client. This may be achieved simply by talking about the weather or their journey. Such exchanges have the effect of making the client feel welcome and at ease. In later sessions, this initial joining should develop into a trusting relationship, achieved through the ability to empathise with the client. Empathy is described in the *Oxford English Dictionary* as the 'power of projecting one's personality into (and so fully comprehending) the object of contemplation'. In other words, seeing and feeling the situation from the client's perspective.

The next step is, through careful conversation, to gain as full a picture as possible of the client's life, general background and development and to establish the exact nature of the 'presenting' problem. This enables the present difficulties to be placed in perspective and the counsellor may then be able to facilitate change if necessary.

## The Building of Confidence

When counselling the visually impaired, all of the above strategies still apply. However, certain other techniques may be usefully employed, and some of the normal rules of counselling may occasionally, and with discretion, have to be broken. It is usually recommended that no physical contact should take place between client and counsellor; this would create a bond between them, thereby engendering a less professional relationship. To expect a newly blind person to speak to a disembodied voice in an unfamiliar and perhaps alien room, is going to destroy the confidence which has enabled them to come to see you in the first place. Allowing the client to take your hand gives orientation, the courage to speak and a sense of security.

Tears often flow, particularly in the first few
sessions. These very tears may often be the cause of
further distress; people – men especially – may be
ashamed of crying. Indeed clients in a post-opera-
tive condition, or suffering from certain disorders,
may have a stinging pain caused by the tears themselves. Alternatively, certain clients may be unable
to shed tears, although they are crying. This too
promotes great pain. It is essential that every counsellor of the visually impaired be aware of these
possibilities.

*Caroline's Story*
There are occasions when there is very little that
the counsellor can do, except be there, for and with
the client. My last interview with Caroline illus-
trates a time when there was no place for words,
but where silence and physical contact gave the
needed support.

Caroline became seriously ill with a severe blood
disorder and as a result she started to lose her
sight. Her husband left her because he was unable
to deal with blindness. Their daughter was very
close to her mother and stayed at home to look
after her. As Caroline's eye condition deteriorated,
she came for counselling. On receipt of her medical
notes, I realised there was no treatment for her
condition. All I could do in subsequent weeks was
to keep her as buoyant as possible whilst occasionally giving support to the daughter. I suggested to

the daughter that she should contact her father and make him aware that the situation was worsening. This she did, and it helped Caroline's morale.

The day came when Caroline was brought in to see me at her own urgent request. As she entered the room, I quickly realised there was something very wrong; she was too tired to speak to me. We sat opposite each other as usual and I held her hand. As I did so, I had a strong conviction that she was dying and I moved my chair beside hers. Still in total silence, I put my other arm around her shoulders and cuddled her. We sat like that for a whole hour until her daughter collected her. Her daughter later told me that as they had left the building, Caroline managed to say that she felt very ill. Shortly afterwards, she collapsed and was admitted to hospital, where she died. Although as a counsellor I had felt ineffectual, I later learned that the counselling sessions had been deeply appreciated both by Caroline and her daughter.

## Making Progress

It is essential to gain as much information as possible from the client about their eye condition, even though medical notes may be available. *The client's own understanding of the situation is what the counsellor needs to work with.* This means that any development is jointly negotiated and the client owns the outcome of any counselling session, and

not just the problem. The responsibility for any
progress, and the credit for it, remains firmly with
the client.

The information sought may relate to what the
client can see in varying light conditions, what
name has been put on the condition and how long
they have been suffering from it. It is also useful to
know how the client became aware of their eye
condition and their initial reaction. This reaction is
likely to be much more profound and have far-
reaching consequences if they have been told in an
insensitive manner, which may lead to greater difficulty in acceptance.

Equally important is to know how the people
around them have reacted, and the degree of
support which has been offered, both by family
and by professionals. Lastly and very importantly,
it is the establishment, in the client's own words, of
the exact nature of the problem for which they are
seeking counselling.

## Areas to Explore

In all counselling, there are three main areas of
knowledge which need to be explored. These are:

- The social history of the client
- The religious background, if any
- The developmental history from childhood.

An understanding of these areas is especially important when counselling the visually impaired. These three main areas are exemplified below in the cases of Millie, Nayana and Albert.

## Millie's Story

When counselling elderly people, which is likely to be the bulk of the work, because 75% of blind and partially sighted people are over the age of 60, it is necessary to have a knowledge of the social changes in this country during the past century. There are people whose minds are active when their sight has completely gone who are now between 80 and 100 years old.

One example of this is Millie, a spinster lady of great dignity, who is now in her mid nineties. She told me in very hushed tones, because she is very proud, that when she and her sister arrived home from school on a Friday, their mother would have no money left for food. To give them a good hot meal, she put broken-up stale bread into a basin with salt and pepper and poured boiling water on it. This was known as 'kettle broth', a warming and sustaining dish familiar to poor people in the early years of the century.

These days, any parent offering such a dish to their child might be considered uncaring. To Millie, it showed how much her parents did care, because, despite the fact that there was no money, her parents had still provided for her. A counsellor unaware of the social difficulties during the time of Millie's childhood might not have understood that this meal was symbolic of that care.

From time to time, a client with a severe visual impairment will come to a counsellor and present the problem as if it is one of sight. Yet after several sessions, it becomes clear that the real problem is something more fundamental which has been exacerbated by the sight loss. Occasionally the person is of a different ethnic origin, and therefore the cultural background is completely different from that in which they are now living. In such cases, it is very important that the counsellor should understand at least the more well-known religious beliefs.

*Nayana's Story*
Nayana, which means 'one with eyes which are a delight to see', was born into a strict Buddhist family in the Far East. Ironically, she was later diagnosed as suffering from a serious and painful eye condition related to Arthritis Uveitis. When this was discovered, she was rejected by her family, as she could not meet their high expectations in terms of academic achievement.

As soon as possible, the family arranged a marriage for Nayana by asking the Buddhist priest for a suitable son-in-law. The priest found a young man whose horoscope matched that of Nayana's father and he was considered to be a good match. Despite Nayana's unhappiness with this arrangement, she was married to him and they came to England. Following the birth of a daughter, her husband began to beat them both. Nayana left him and tried to fend for herself. She had no money, as she had lost her job because of her eye condition. Despite her difficulties, she managed successfully to bring up her daughter, who subsequently attended university.

Very lonely, and in a state of despair, Nayana met a strong, young, ill-educated white man, who told her she was beautiful. The relationship became sordid and at that point she sought counselling. Although the eye condition was her presenting case, it quickly became clear that she was in a dangerous situation and this was now her main difficulty. The eye condition had dictated the course of her whole life, but it was apparent that she needed help and counselling in wider fields.

## The Religious Dimension

In our multicultural society, the counsellor will encounter – and needs to have some knowledge of – a wide variety of creeds, customs and denominations of the major religious faiths. Clearly this is necessary in order to be equipped to help those who profess to, or have come to reject, these faiths. In Nayana's case the understanding of her background was very important in the counselling sessions – another such client is Thomas.

## Thomas's Story

At the age of 15, Thomas was told that owing to an inherited eye condition, he would never be able to drive a car; his sight was unlikely to improve as he matured and it might even deteriorate. His turbulent feelings at this news led to his truancy from school and bad behaviour at home. His mother took him to see the priest at the local church which Thomas had been attending since his baptism. With great kindness, but total lack of understanding, the priest simply said, 'You are in God's hands and must pray.'

This did nothing to console Thomas and his continued bad behaviour led to him being brought to the centre where I work. Having had a teenage son of my own, I knew what he was suffering. After a few weeks, Thomas and I became good friends. He went back to school, joined in the school's musical production and did well in his exams. Thomas then went to university, where he gained a degree in theology and was ordained as a minister in a non-conformist church. He has accepted the fact that he will never drive a car, but intends one day to employ his own chauffeur!

## Lydia's Story

Not so straightforward is the case of Lydia, who is

widowed and now lives alone. With a very strong faith, she has accepted the macular degeneration which has badly damaged her sight, remaining dignified and ladylike. However, she is continually hurt by the seeming indifference shown to her by the members of her church congregation. She has a car to take her to the service and when she is sitting waiting for it to collect her afterwards, people pass her by without speaking, intent instead on what they are saying to each other. She has no eye contact with them and they act as if she isn't there, which makes her feel invisible and very lonely (see Chapter 1 for more on the significance of loss of eye contact).

## Insights from Psychology

Thanks to the work of psychologists such as Erikson and Winnicott, we acquired in the second half of the twentieth century a much fuller understanding of the important influence of child development upon later life. In this connection, the traumatic effect of the birth experience is now understood; and it is widely held that the severance of the umbilical cord causes a sense of loss and anxiety in the newly born child.

Then very soon three new bonds between the child and the mother are created. The first is the cord of touch, with the mother cuddling, loving and feeding the baby, giving acceptance and sustenance. The second is the cord of sight, which develops through eye contact between the mother and child; this occurs much earlier than was at one time believed and leads to a sense of security. The third is a bond of trust and faith, which develops gradually out of the cord of sight, enabling the child to know that if mother leaves she will return. The role of the father is now seen as much more significant, from the infant's earliest days, than used to be thought.

Thus the child gains a feeling of belonging, of having a place or status in the world, which in itself gives a sense of achievement. Already we have the beginnings of a dynamic cycle which is the normal pattern of most people's lives. Acceptance by those around us will go on to sustain us, giving us a status in society where we will be able to achieve and gain acceptance by a wider circle of people. Two cases here will illustrate the benefit of the dynamic cycle and the tragic consequences of its reversal.

## The Blind Baby

Great care has to be taken when a child is born without sight. The mother's voice becomes even more important, as the auditory contact replaces the cord of sight. The child without sight needs to find out where he is by flailing his arms around to discover what his world is like. Distressing though it may be to watch, it is essential that the child should be allowed to behave in this way. Once the parents have got over the initial shock and have had sympathetic counselling and practical help, a loving but not over-protective environment can be created and parents' attitudes may then become totally positive.

A well-known correspondent and presenter of various programmes for the BBC describes in his autobiography how he and his brother, also blind from birth, greatly appreciate the attitude of their parents, who were positive and loving. They focused on their education and upbringing, to the point where both brothers became very successful in their chosen careers and have been able to lead full and happy lives.

## Albert's Story

On the other hand, Albert, born in 1918 to a young unmarried girl, was born blind, taken away from his mother immediately and has been in institutions all his life. He has never had a home. He has never owned anything other than a few clothes and he has just gone into the last place he is likely to live in, a retirement home for the elderly blind. He has no family, no love, no money, no possessions, no confidence, is very frail and has had poor health all his life.

Albert found it difficult to tell me how he has never felt he has had a place in society. He has always been on the outside, and took my hand to

give himself the security to say what he wanted
to tell me. I noticed his grip was firm as he
steadied himself emotionally; this belied his very
frail, quiet voice, which he told me later is due
to his bad nerves. Distressing as it was to
witness the exposure of these awful feelings, I felt
it was necessary for him, even at his age, to be
able to feel he had the space and the trust to do
so. How different are the worlds of the successful
and ebullient Peter, who was loved and valued,
and Albert who was abandoned and felt
completely rejected.

In neither of these two cases could there have been
a cord of sight. Despite this, one forged a good
relationship with his parents, which led to acceptance by society and a sense of his own self-worth.
The second case shows what happens when no
bond is created and self-worth does not develop.
The adult then appears to have been completely
rejected by society.

   In Albert's case, the dynamic cycle has gone into
reverse. Rejected by his mother at birth, against all
odds he tried to achieve as he grew up, but in his
situation he got nowhere and had no status in
society. The result was that he has, by living in
institutions all his life, never sustained himself and
still longs to be accepted. The value of the support
of a professional counsellor to Albert and others in
his plight can hardly be over-emphasised – far

more than anti-depressant drugs or sleeping pills (which is all a GP can offer).

## Counselling Family and Friends

Counselling the families of the visually impaired can be of great value. They too are worried and anxious. Their lives also have changed dramatically. Their patience may not be limitless. The sight loss is also the family's loss and consequently bereavement counselling is an appropriate technique to use here as well. Without this greater understanding, families' reactions can often be inappropriate to the needs of the person who has lost, or who is losing, their sight.

*Sheila's Story*
Sheila, a mother of six children by two husbands, suffered two retinal detachments suddenly and unexpectedly, probably caused by the violence sustained in her first marriage. There were many variations in the reactions of family members, from total disbelief and denial by her parents to unquestioning acceptance by her youngest child and an almost suffocating over-protection by her husband.

Sheila herself was absolutely devastated. Initially she came alone for counselling and, because it became evident that the variance in the family's reactions was adding to her distress, after the second interview I suggested she ask her husband to make an appointment with me. He is a very caring man and came the following week. I was now able to deal with his grief and lack of under-standing of his wife's turbulent and unbearable feelings. Worried about the children, whose ages ranged from nineteen to nine, we looked together at their feelings and their own personal loss. Practical means to help their mother were talked through and later carried out.

At the same time, Sheila's husband realised that his over-protectiveness was the result of caring too much. He was doing the things for his wife he would have expected for himself had the situation been reversed and was projecting his own fear on to her. It will take some time for things to become normal again, but we have now reached the point where Sheila comes for support every week and has accepted long cane mobility training.

The following two cases show the long-term effects of over-protection where no counselling has been available. These two cases are also contrasting because of different individual reactions.

*Yvonne's Story*
At the age of 14, Yvonne left home to go and live with a 19-year-old friend, who later married. Yvonne continued to live with the couple after their marriage, and worked until the age of 44, when she found driving difficult and sought an eye

test. The optician sent her to a specialist, who told her that she had the hereditary condition Retinitis Pigmentosa and would eventually lose her sight completely.

At this point, Yvonne went into a clinical depression and was taken into a psychiatric hospital. On her return home, her friends refused to allow her to do anything at all, although at this stage she still had a great deal of residual vision. She made no effort herself and allowed them to take over her life. With their overwhelming but misplaced desire to support her, they have made a rod for their own backs. The point has now been reached where Yvonne's life is a burden to her friends and they would like her to go into a home. Yvonne, however, is resisting, not having the courage to relinquish her cocooned existence.

## Terry's Story

Terry, in his forties, was the victim of a serious road accident, sustaining severe head injuries in which the optic nerve was severed. On recovery he was found to be totally blind, but with no serious brain injury. He was married with two children and when he returned home he was smothered with love and comfort by his wife, children and parents.

Six months later he went to the Rehabilitation and Assessment Centre for the newly blind at Torquay (see Chapter 9: Registration and Afterwards). There it was discovered that Terry could do nothing for himself as a result of their over-protection; he could not even dress himself or shave – he was like a baby. The staff and other residents at the Centre gradually enabled him to do little things for himself until he learned to use a white cane, from which point he began to go into the workshops and join in. After three months, he was able to go with some of the other men each night to a local bar – where it was Terry who played the piano for all the customers. He had reclaimed his old personality by seizing the opportunities offered by rehabilitation to become himself and live life again to the full.

## Gradual Sight Loss

Immediate and total sight loss as in the cases of Sheila and Terry seldom occurs; in most cases it is more gradual. This is an area where the professionally trained counsellor's knowledge of eye conditions comes in. It is sometimes wrongly supposed that gradual loss of sight is not felt or noticed. In some cases the sight goes suddenly onto a lower level and as one person put it to me, she almost heard it deteriorate. 'It was,' she said, 'like being at the opticians where a new lens is put into the frame which is on your face. As it goes into the slot it clicks and that is just how it seems to me each time I go onto a lower level.'

Other people find that to bump into something

with their head – such an easy thing to do when you cannot see where you are going – causes a worsening of the situation; and more serious mishaps or illness cause a further deterioration. These people suffer a series of shocks, beyond the original shock, and some of them will need a counsellor's informed support to deal more positively with the trauma of deteriorating vision until the sight is finally gone – and after.

## Practical Considerations

No matter how well the adjustments are made in most cases, there are continuing feelings of frustration and anger. It is, for instance, humiliating to have personal documents read to you, such as your bank statement and private letters. Whilst you may have nothing to hide, things which are very personal remain so always. To allow someone else to see such things is a great sacrifice, and the person who has to make it feels belittled. Life at times appears to become unreal, 'It is enough to drive you to drink,' as a client once said to me. Other people have said things in a similar vein.

Of course, the majority of people in this situation do adjust; some take longer than others, but most get the welling up of these negative feelings from time to time throughout the rest of their lives. If they have been fortunate enough to see a counsellor at the very beginning, they may be able to

deal with these readjustments as time goes on
without returning for specialist help. However, a
counsellor is most likely to see people when they
have reached a point of depression, often caused by
the initial shock which has not been properly dealt
with.

## The Gift of Sight – A Mixed Blessing

In recent years, as medicine, medical skills and
technology have advanced, it is sometimes possible
to give a person sight when they were born without
it. Operations of this kind are occasionally
performed, with varying degrees of success, on a
number of suitable people. The world applauds the
surgeons who have been given the skills to perform
these sight-giving miracles. There is much publicity
and everyone feels good, not only because of its
rarity, but because it brings with it a sense of relief
to the sighted, who themselves fear blindness.

The trauma which follows these 'miraculous'
operations, however, is seldom publicised. Some
patients, particularly children, adjust, although it
may take time. To many, the experience is unbe-
lievably frightening and some find that what they
have never been able to see before makes it impossible for them to walk about without closing their
eyes. They have no spatial awareness, and words
like 'height, width, depth' are meaningless.

People's faces, whilst all different, can be so

incongruous as to be beyond belief, and light itself, of course, is a great shock. The height of anything above their reach, such as buildings, double-decker buses, trees and particularly the sky, can be a source of terror. Just imagine what it must be like to stand at the foot of a mountain and keep looking up until you see its peak, when you have no built-in equipment to imagine such a thing. A few people have been so traumatised that they have been known to take their own lives.

For counsellors for blind people, the first need is to understand the trauma of going from a familiar world into an unfamiliar one: the trauma experienced by going from darkness into light is no less nor more dramatic than going from light into darkness. Each is equally frightening. But whereas the rare 'miracle' hits the headlines, sight loss does not, on the whole, stimulate the public to imaginative awareness or empathy. Well-meaning but misguided remarks may be the reverse of helpful, and embarrassed avoidance is a frequent reaction that leaves blind people feeling alone and desolate in a colourless, hazard-strewn world.

It is, as we have seen, the role and privilege of the counsellor, drawing on the knowledge and insights gained in professional training, to give the support which will enable the client to become more secure and confident in facing the future.

# 9

# *Registration and Afterwards*

## Registration

The World Health Organisation provides a simple yardstick which can indicate how much or how little sight a person has, when registration as blind or partially sighted is suggested:

If a person is able to see fingers raised at face level 20 feet away but no further, they are eligible for registration as partially sighted. If a person is able to see fingers raised at face level 10 feet away but no further, they are eligible for registration as blind.

Anyone who has reached the point where they suspect, or have been told, that they ought to consider registration, may need to be reassured about what registration entails.

(a) Registration is voluntary. No one can be compelled to ask for it, and it will not mean that they will be 'labelled', or investigated, or considered unable to live independently.

(b) Registration follows a detailed eye examination by a consultant ophthalmologist, who will measure the precise activity of vision in each eye. If he or she so advises, there is a long (very long!) form, BD8, to be filled in by the consultant, copies of which are sent to the patient, their GP, Social Services and to a government body concerned with population statistics.

(c) The advantage of being registered either as blind or partially sighted is that it opens the door to whatever practical – from Social Services initially – or financial help may be available. The law concerning the latter, dealing with tax relief and some modest care allowance, has changed in recent years. The only long-established relief given to blind people is a reduction off a TV licence.

(d) Help is available to people who are registered through a specialist organisation, such as the Partially Sighted Society and the Retinitis Pigmentosa Society, and other societies for specific conditions. Being in touch with those bodies may not only reduce feelings of isolation, but also provide useful information about the specific eye condition.

## Getting Help

Once registration is in progress, the patient and their relatives may well leave the hospital suffering from shock, having been told little or nothing about what their next step should be. In many cases, the names of the big national organisations for the blind may come to mind – the RNIB, for instance – and it is useful to mention at this point an excellent handbook published by that organisation, entitled *You and Your Sight*, which answers many of the basic questions. (See page 163 for further details about this book and where to obtain it). However, the next source of information and help in the process of registration is the local Social Services department, who should have received their copy of the form BD8.

## Social Services

It is the statutory duty of the Social Services department to make contact, by sending a social worker to discuss all aspects of registration, in order to confirm the patient's agreement to registration, and to discuss what practical help may be needed and what is on offer. High on the list of priorities will be the question of some form of mobility training, notably in the use of the long white cane for those who would benefit from it. Unfortunately, such training must be carried out by specialist social workers, of whom there are far too few to cover adequately the needs of those waiting for, or undergoing, training in some localities.

There is hope that the situation will improve because of arrangements suggested by the Guide Dogs Association. Their regulations require that no application for ownership of a guide dog can be considered without proper mobility training with a white cane; they have therefore offered to supplement the training Social Services already provide, sending their own specialist mobility officers into the community. This would surely benefit many people who are newly registered, and give them the opportunity to apply later on for assessment for training with a guide dog.

*Local Voluntary Organisations*
In addition to contact with Social Services, further practical 'hands-on' help will be needed in most cases. This is to be found in the local voluntary associations, about which Social Services can supply information. Many are registered charities, depending on donations and on the knowledge and help supplied by local people. They cannot afford to employ many paid staff and depend largely on volunteer help. Their committees are likely to include some blind people, and each body will decide where they feel the greatest needs lie in their own district. In some instances, where they co-operate with the Social Services department, they receive a small grant allocated by the Social Services Committee, which is reviewed annually. Many of these societies have some link with the local hospital, perhaps through the presence of an ophthalmic surgeon on the committee.

The activities and types of help offered by local

societies vary widely, according to assessment of
need and the funds available, and urban societies
differ from rural ones. However, some of the
following (though certainly not all in any one
locality) will most likely be found:

- Transport to and from the centre
- A lunch club, one or more days a week
- Teaching of movement to music and yoga (these
  improve the condition of the joints)
- Dancing (part of mobility training, using orienta-
  tion skills and giving confidence in space)
- Teaching of touch typing, Braille and Moon
- Daily living skills, including cooking (especially
  useful for men living alone) and mobility in the
  home
- Advice about useful gadgets
- Pottery, and art and crafts classes
- Hairdressing, for men and women, on a regular
  basis
- A weekly 'shop' stocked from a non profit-
  making trade supplier
- Visiting clothes shops with racks of new clothes
  for sale
- Outings, sometimes even including holidays at
  home and abroad
- Celebratory meals (as at Christmas)
- Speakers and entertainers.

Of considerable importance are the various social

groups which meet regularly to enjoy common interests such as music, quizzes and crosswords, bingo and gardening. Out-of-town centres, with greater distances and expense in bringing people together, may meet less often; their pursuits may include ramblings, with a pub lunch, tandem-riding (with a sighted person in front) and possibly riding for the disabled.

Equally important in town or country, is the availability of someone to read a letter or help with filling in a form, as well as legal and financial advisers.

One local society at least – and there may be more – has a care line in operation, whereby every member on the centre's list is telephoned regularly to make sure all is well. And, rarely till now but much needed and appreciated, counselling may be available for visually impaired people and their families.

Most local societies produce and send out tapes regularly, containing articles from the local newspaper and other items of interest. Information may be available on tape about events in the area – concerts, theatres, etc. – and other tapes may be produced for football fans.

What I believe is lacking – and is seriously needed – is one national help line for *all* registered blind people (similar to those of the motoring organisations) which would link them to services available in their locality.

# The National Societies

Information, advice and instructions are freely available from the national societies listed below. This information is produced on request in several different formats: printed pamphlets (in large print if required), on audio tape or sometimes in Braille. An initial telephone call, on the lines indicated below, will provide the contact needed. These charities, set up for the benefit of blind people, have grown tremendously and have their own specialities, though their roles have overlapped to some extent (this is due to laws governing charities, which prevent donated money from being used for any purpose other than that for which it was given).

The major national societies in the field of blindness are:

- The Royal National Institute for the Blind (RNIB)
- Action for Blind People (ABP)
- The Guide Dogs for the Blind Association (GDBA)
- St Dunstan's
- The National Talking Newspaper and Magazine Service (TNA-UK)
- The National Library for the Blind.

*The Royal National Institute for the Blind (RNIB)*
This is the leading charity for blind people. The

RNIB has a considerable amount of influence in the fields of law-making and social welfare, and produces a wide range of pamphlets to publicise its extensive services.

The RNIB plays a major part in the education of visually impaired people, from infancy to college and beyond, including training in Braille and Moon. It is active in the areas of employment services, leisure activities including some care homes and holiday venues, and advice on financial and legal matters and on housing. Attention is drawn here to three of the RNIB's many publications, and how they may be obtained.

*You and Your Sight* by Hilary Todd and Francesca Wolf, HMSO, £4.95. The book can be ordered direct from RNIB Customer Services, PO Box 173, Peterborough PE2 6WS. Telephone 0845 7023153 (at local call rates).

*Your Guide to the RNIB* is a clear and comprehensive guide to what is available in the association's fields of operation. It gives addresses and telephone numbers for the offices in London, Scotland and Northern Ireland, as well as telephone numbers for specialist services and advice. To obtain this guide, call the RNIB on 0845 7669999.

*The RNIB Catalogue of Products* is also obtainable by calling 0207 388 1266. It is very large, and lists a huge range of items for work, leisure and daily living for blind people of all ages. The catalogue is offered free of charge, though a donation towards the production cost (£4) is appreciated. Items listed for sale in it are at cost price and carry no VAT if bought for people who are registered.

*The Talking Book Service* is a much valued part of the RNIB. There are over 11,000 books to choose from, and every year some 450 titles are added; books are specially read by professionals and recorded unabridged, including fiction and non-fiction, books for children and some in Asian languages and in Welsh. Books are sent by freepost. For more information, telephone 0845 7023153.

*The RNIB Cassette Library* has over 18,000 titles, including text books, works of reference, student editions of fiction and a Braille library of more than 70,000 volumes.

*RNIB Manor House, Skills Development Centre*
The Centre caters specifically for those aged between 18 and 65, who have become severely visually impaired. For information about Manor House, contact the nearest Job Centre, and ask for an appointment with the Disability Employment Adviser, mentioning that you want to find out about Manor House, Skills Development Centre at Torquay. In cases where there is a dual disability, you should contact your local Social Services department. Those whose disability will prevent them from continuing to work, should also contact Social Services.

An important point to bear in mind is that your

local Social Services department will need to fund
the assessment that Manor House will carry out on
your first visit, in addition to any further training
and living accommodation that the Centre will
offer.

If you would like further information, contact
RNIB, Manor House, Middle Lincoln Road,
Torquay TQ1 2NG. The telephone number is
01803 214523.

## Action for Blind People (ABP)

This charity began in 1857 as the Surrey
Association for the General Welfare of the Blind. In
1876 it was renamed the South London Association
for the Blind, and it was the first organisation to
employ blind women. In 1910 it became the
London Association for the Blind, continuing to
provide workshops for blind people. Such large
orders were placed with these workshops from 1914
onwards by the Army and the Royal Navy, that the
financial rewards enabled the Association to open
many more workshops in the London area. By 1923
they were the largest institution in the world to
employ blind women. By 1945 they were able to
open Swail House at Epsom, a purpose-built
complex which includes accommodation for blind
people.

ABP is now a national organisation and in 1991
reflected this in yet another change of name,
becoming Action for Blind People. It specialises in

training people to staff their workshops for the blind, but also maintains an interest in other aspects of blind welfare and gives general advice.

ABP produce a tape-recording called 'Getting On'. This gives information on a whole range of subjects, including the availability of statutory and voluntary services, registration and entitlement to benefit. They also try to work closely with the local voluntary services for the blind and are anxious to develop relationships with hospitals. This is part of their endeavour to offer a service at the point of diagnosis of irreversible sight loss.

ABP also run a limited number of care homes for the elderly blind in various parts of the country, and they provide some holiday venues, particularly in the South of England.

For information about all their services, telephone their London hotline on 0207 732 8771.

## The Guide Dogs for the Blind Association (GDBA)

This organisation was set up in England during the late 1920s and is now nationwide. GDBA has 15 training centres, including seven main regional ones, for the purpose of breeding and training dogs, and running courses for blind people to teach them to use a guide dog efficiently and safely, for work, leisure and companionship. GDBA employs fully trained rehabilitation officers, who teach the use of the long cane in order to give the confidence needed to go on and train with a dog. Guide dog owners become expert dog-handlers; everyone who applies for a guide dog is considered, and no one is turned down because they have insufficient money.

GDBA continues to support both dog and owner throughout their time together, even when the dog is retired. The organisation also has two hotels for the use of guide dog owners with their dog and family or friends, so that they can have a holiday together.

GDBA have been pioneers in their field, and their advice is sought on all aspects of their work by organisations in many countries. Their contact telephone number is 01189 835555.

## *St Dunstan's*

St Dunstan's cares for men and women of the armed forces who have lost their sight in the service of their country, whether in war or peace. It was founded in 1915 and took its name from a house so named in Regents Park, which was lent to the organisation. It provides rehabilitation and employment skills, training, medical care and housing for St Dunstaners and their families, widows and widowers. They also maintain a nursing, residential and training centre at Ovingdean, Brighton. St Dunstan's administers a Trust – the Diana Gubbay Trust for the Blind – which provides assistance to ex-members of the forces whose blindness is not due to their military service.

Occasionally St Dunstan's has extended its assistance to members of the police and fire services who have suffered sight loss as a result of their public duty. They can be reached on 0207 723 5021.

## The National Talking Newspaper and Magazine Service (TNA-UK)

This is a charity which provides high-quality recordings on cassette – and some on computer formats – for people with impaired vision. For an annual subscription of £25 (£35 overseas) members are allowed as many titles as they can enjoy. Cassettes on offer include national and Sunday papers and a wide range of magazines, including *Radio Times* and *TV Times*.

The telephone number of the service is 01435 866102.

## The National Library for the Blind

The library offers Braille books, which may be borrowed free of charge via the postal services.

Their contact phone number is 0161 355 2000.

## Telephoning – Directory Inquiries

It is good for blind people to maintain their independence from sighted help where possible. Once registered as blind, they are entitled to free use of Directory Enquiries; an initial call to the British

Telecom number 195 will lead to their being given a PIN number and through it access to numbers without further charge.

## The Disability Discrimination Act

The main areas covered by this act (listed by the RNIB) are as follows:

- Getting goods and services
- Getting and keeping a job
- Using public transport
- Buying or renting a flat or house.

The RNIB produces a simple, useful booklet on this Act, with examples of how it may serve to reduce discrimination against blind and partially sighted people.

You can contact the RNIB on 0345 669999 – for the price of a local call – for further information.

# Index

Numbers in **bold** indicate Figures.